BASIC NURSING PROCEDURES

BASIC NURSING PROCEDURES

GRACE V. HORNEMANN, BA, RN

10 9 8

LIBRARY OF CONGRESS CATALOG CARD NUMBER: 77-094835
ISBN: 0-8273-1320-9

Printed in the United States of America
Published simultaneously in Canada
by Nelson Canada,
A Division of International Thomson Limited

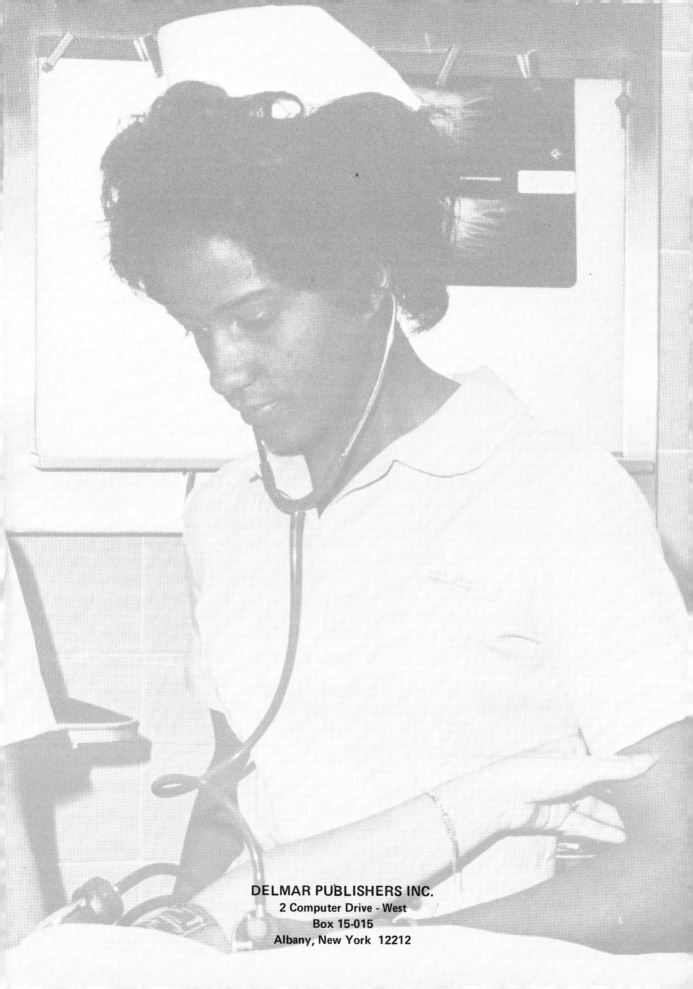

DELMAR PUBLISHERS INC.
2 Computer Drive - West
Box 15-015
Albany, New York 12212

PREFACE

Basic Nursing Procedures was written to provide the beginning student with the basic skills needed to perform bedside nursing care. By studying the skills presented, both the nurse assistant and practical nurse can benefit from the use of this text. The procedures are arranged so that the more difficult skills are covered later — after fundamental skills have been mastered. Also, each section can be studied independently of the others. This allows the instructor to present the material as it best suits the particular class of students. The procedures described may vary among different health care facilities. The location, size, and type of facility will influence the choice of methods and the equipment used.

Although disposable items have become part of the standard equipment for some facilities, the student should learn to perform procedures without depending on disposables exclusively. This belief is reflected by references to the care of nondisposable items whenever it was felt such items might still be used. The author, when necessary, has tried to present the advantages of using one technique or piece of equipment over another. Rather than stressing variations in method, emphasis has been placed on the *principles* of nursing care; these are shown in bold type. The procedures illustrate and reinforce these principles.

Each unit uses a similar format. The procedure is broken down into steps. Important points to be remembered — in boldface type — immediately follow each related step. Behavioral objectives at the beginning of each unit help the student establish goals for learning the information presented. A vocabulary section, suggested activities, and questions follow each unit to help the student review small amounts of material at a time. Self-evaluations follow each of the twelve major sections and test student ability to retain and apply a larger volume of information.

The value of the nurse-patient relationship is stressed throughout *Basic Nursing Procedures*. Ways in which the nurse may show consideration and concern for the patient are suggested. It is well known that the practical nurse may be required to gradually assume more responsibility in day-to-day contacts with the patient, but it must always be remembered that *no procedure should be undertaken unless the student has been taught and is authorized to do it under the direction of a registered nurse or physician.*

The author, Grace V. Hornemann, is a graduate of St. Vincent's Hospital School of Nursing, New York City. She received a baccalaureate degree and continued with graduate studies in nursing education at the School of Education, New York University. Mrs. Hornemann is qualified to teach Special Education as well as Nursing.

Other Delmar publications for the practical nurse and related health careers are:

Body Structures and Functions — E. Ferris and E. Skelley
Obstetrics for the Nurse — B. Anderson and P. Shapiro
Microbiology for Health Careers — E. Ferris
Geriatrics: A Study of Maturity — E. Caldwell and B. Hegner

CONTENTS

SECTION VI MAINTAINING THE PATIENT'S SAFETY AND COMFORT

SECTION VII THE PATIENT'S PERSONAL HYGIENE

SECTION VIII ASEPTIC TECHNIQUES

SECTION IX APPLICATIONS OF HEAT AND COLD

SECTION X RESPIRATORY, EYE AND EAR TREATMENTS

SECTION XI THERAPEUTIC PROCEDURES FOR THE EXCRETORY SYSTEM

SECTION XII CARING FOR PATIENTS WITH SPECIAL NEEDS

SECTION I BASIC CONCEPTS AND HEALTH PRACTICES

unit 1 the health team

OBJECTIVES

After studying this unit, the student will be able to:

- List members of the health team.
- Explain the functions of each member of the health team.

Care of the sick, the prevention of illness and the promotion of health and general welfare requires a combination of knowledge and skills; more than one person can provide. A group of professionally trained persons is needed. The nurse is one of a group — referred to as the health team — who contributes skills and expertise to promote the health and general welfare. Each member of the team must understand and respect the contributions of the other members. Nursing is a cooperative profession.

HEALTH TEAM MEMBERS

The health team may include the following persons; each is especially taught to perform certain skills:

- The *physician* makes the medical diagnosis and prescribes medication, treatment, diet, and limits on activity. All X-ray and laboratory studies are ordered by the physician.

- The *registered nurse*, RN, coordinates patient's care with the functions of the other team members. She interprets and carries out the orders of the doctor. She plans the nursing care around the needs of the patient.

- The *licensed practical* or *licensed vocational nurse*, LPN/LVN, gives bedside care under the supervision of the registered nurse and/or the doctor. The LPN/LVN performs many treatments and gives medications if supervised and taught to do so.

- The *nurse assistant* provides personal bedside care and helps the RN or LPN when necessary. Other duties include collecting specimens, feeding patient, and responding to call signals, lifting the patient, and escorting patients to X-ray or laboratory department.

- The *physical therapist* takes part in restoring the use of muscle function through heat, cold, pressure, massage, exercise and manipulation. The patient's re-education is a vital part of the work.

- The *pharmacist* prepares the drugs prescribed by the physician.

- The *dietitian* plans special diets with the proper proportion of food elements as prescribed by the physician.

- The *occupational therapist* instructs the patient in diversions and occupations which he is able to perform during convalescence. Occupational therapy is a vital part of the care given to patients with a long-term (chronic) illness.

- The *social worker* counsels and advises the patient about problems associated with the illness. With a knowledge of various agencies, the social worker can help the patient with financial, social, and other personal problems.

- The *technician* is skilled in performing procedures which are specific to an area of care; for example, analysis of specimens, taking of X rays, operating room techniques, and inhalation therapy.

- The *auxiliary workers* include those in food service, central supply, housekeeping and others who help in the maintenance and function of the hospital facilities.

In those health-related facilities where the physician's assistant and the nurse practitioner are involved with patient care, they, too, are considered members of the health team.

- The *physician's assistant* is a new career. After an extensive course of study, the physician's assistant may participate in patient care by taking histories, doing physical examinations, and ordering laboratory studies, all under the supervision of a medical doctor. Duties also may include helping the physician by applying casts and suturing minor cuts.

- The *nurse practitioner* role is often confused with that of the physician's assistant. Nurse practitioners, however, are required to have an RN license and nursing experience before entering the special program which prepares them to provide primary health care. Unlike the physician's assistant, the nurse practitioner views the patient through the eyes of a nurse, focusing on meeting the basic needs and treating the health problems.

HOSPITAL ORGANIZATION

The hospital organization becomes more complex with the expansion of the health team and health services. As the organization grows, the need for the various departments to work together becomes more important. The patient is the central focus and major concern at each level. Within each department,

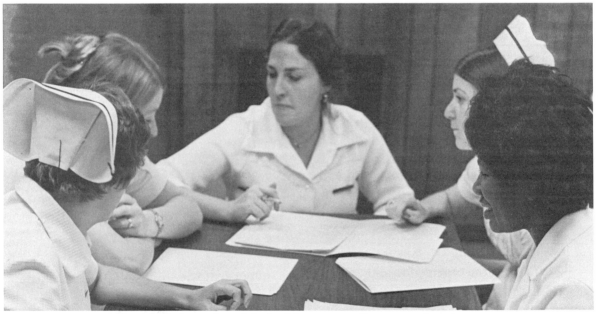

Fig. 1-1 Each member of the health team contributes to a plan of care.

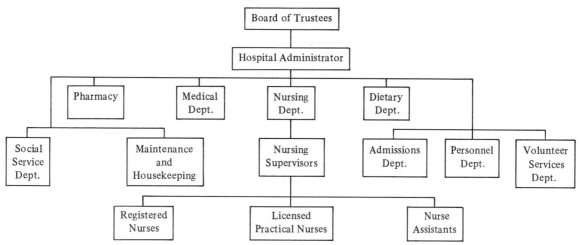

Fig. 1-2 Health team members form part of the hospital organization

the patient is the center of the planning and decision making which takes place.

SPECIALIZATION

Scientific and medical advances have led to specialization for both the physician and the nurse. Diagnosis is often done by a team of physicians. Each one is a specialist in a certain disease or part of the human body. Many surgeons for example, perform only certain types of operations.

There is a constant increase in the number of nurses who undertake advanced study in some special field of interest such as maternal and child health, intensive care nursing and public health nursing. As specialization increases, the nurse's ability to get along with co-workers, patients, and others becomes more important.

VOCABULARY

• Define the following words

auxiliary	dietition	occupational therapist
chronic	episodic	physical therapist
coordinate	health history	specialist
convalescence	inhalation	therapy
diagnosis	manipulation	

SUGGESTED ACTIVITIES

• Prepare a report for the class on one member of the health team. Include in your report the type of education needed, various specialists in the field, and the general duties. List the ways each member helps others in the health team. Choose a member of the health team outside of the nursing profession.

• Prepare a report for the class on the duties of the practical nurse in a specialized field. Include any advanced training which is required. You may want to investigate one of the following specialties:

Medical-surgical   Geriatrics
Pediatrics   Psychiatric
Obstetrics

REVIEW

A. Give an example of the duties performed by each of the following members of the health team.

1. Practical/vocational nurse

2. Physical therapist

3. Nurse Assistant

4. Technician

5. Social Worker

B. Briefly answer the following questions.

1. Describe the way the health team concept avoids problems which might arise from specialization.

2. List three services provided by auxiliary workers in the hospital.

3. What is the role of the registered nurse?

4. Who is the focus of all departments in the hospital organization?

5. What is the health team?

unit 2 the licensed practical nurse

OBJECTIVES

After studying this unit, the student will be able to:

- Define the role of the practical nurse.
- List the organizations which set standards for accreditation.
- List ways to keep informed about nursing matters.

The licensed practical nurse, through education and clinical experience, obtains knowledge, skill and judgment. With these abilities and under the direction of a registered nurse, doctor, or dentist, the LPN provides patient care. Continued education prepares the LPN to assume more complex responsibilities. She can also obtain education and experience to work in a special field like maternity nursing, pediatrics, and care of the aged.

BEDSIDE NURSING

Practical nurses make a noteworthy contribution to the health care of the nation. Licensed practical nurses can give most of the bedside care that is needed safely and efficiently. Bedside nursing is the most important aspect of the practical nurse's duties. In addition to attending to the patient's personal needs, the duties include providing a comfortable environment by adjusting lights, ventilating the room, and keeping the noise level down. Food should be served promptly. Drugs and treatment should be given as ordered by the doctor. Nursing care may involve bathing the patient, changing the linens, positioning the patient, and using modern equipment. All bedside nursing requires careful judgment.

THE LPN AS A TEAM MEMBER

The nurse spends a great deal of time

with the patient. The nurse, as a result of great time spent with the patient, has the singular opportunity to help the patient understand the cooperation needed among health team members. By observing the way

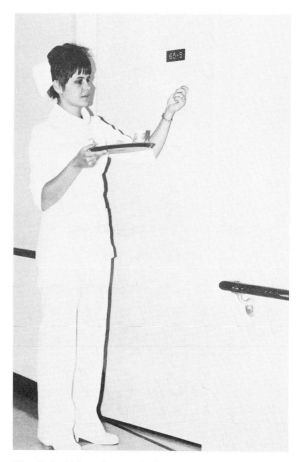

Fig. 2-1 Education and clinical experience prepare the licensed practical nurse to accept responsibility such as giving medications.

Code of Ethics
for the Licensed Practical / Vocational Nurse

The Licensed Practical/Vocational Nurse shall:

1. Consider as a basic obligation the conservation of life and the prevention of disease.

2. Promote and protect the physical, mental, emotional, and spiritual health of the patient and his family.

3. Fulfill all duties faithfully and efficiently.

4. Function within established legal guidelines.

5. Accept personal responsibility (for his acts) and seek to merit the respect and confidence of all members of the health team.

6. Hold in confidence all matters coming to his knowledge, in the practice of his profession, and in no way and at no time violate this confidence.

7. Give conscientious service and charge just remuneration.

8. Learn and respect the religious and cultural beliefs of his patient and of all people.

9. Meet his obligation to the patient by keeping abreast of current trends in health care through reading and continuing education.

10. As a citizen of the United States of America, uphold the laws of the land and seek to promote legislation which shall meet the health needs of its people.

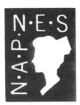 National Association for Practical Nurse Education and Service, Inc.

122 East 42nd Street, New York, N.Y. 10017

Fig. 2-2 A code of ethics provides guidance in performing nursing care.

the patient acts with his family and friends, the nurse may feel that there is need for a social worker or chaplain. By reporting her observations to the RN, the practical nurse can help schedule care to allow the patient time for meeting with the social worker, the physical therapist, the X-ray technician, and other health team members. Everyone needs the cooperation of other health team members. The patient's trust in the health care being given will depend greatly on the cooperation of everyone involved in his care.

NURSING ORGANIZATIONS

When a student practical nurse has completed a course in an accredited school, he/she is eligible to take the examination for licensure given by the state. Licensure exists for the protection of the patient and the nurse. Completion of an accredited program and passing the state board examinations are necessary for licensure to practice.

In an ever-advancing vocation such as practical nursing, it is necessary to keep up with the new techniques, policies, and practices. It is also necessary to know about laws and regulations which affect nurses and nursing. This can be done by reading professional journals and participating in the nursing organizations. There are local, state, and national organizations.

The national nursing organizations which affect practical nursing are:

- National League for Nursing (NLN)
- National Association for Practical Nurse Education and Service (NAPNES)
- National Federation of Licensed Practical Nurses (NFLPN)

National League for Nursing. The main objective of this organization is to maintain and improve standards of nursing education. It is made up of many councils which represent professional, technical, and practical nursing and the different educational programs offered. Through testing, the NLN helps schools to select qualified students. It takes an active part in accrediting programs for practical nursing as well as registered nursing. Its official magazine is the *American Journal of Nursing (AJN)*.

The National Association for Practical Nurse Education and Service, Inc. This is the oldest practical nurse organization. It has given valuable leadership and promoted setting educational standards for the accreditation of schools of practical nursing. NAPNES developed the code of ethics (see figure 2-2) and promotes voluntary continuing education programs for practical nurses. The *Journal of Practical Nursing* is the official magazine. Membership consists of other interested personnel besides practical nurses.

The National Federation of Licensed Practical Nurses (NFLPN). This national organization was established in 1949 for licensed practical nurses. It sponsors workshops and seminars, which can be used for continuing education credits. *Nursing Care* is the official magazine.

Both national practical nurse organizations (NAPNES and NFLPN) work toward the betterment of practical nurse education and service.

VOCABULARY

- Define the following words

accreditation	legislation	standard
conscientious	licensure	technique

continuing education	remuneration	vocation
cooperation	seminar	workshop

SUGGESTED ACTIVITIES

- Find out what benefits can be obtained from membership in the Licensed Practical Nurses Association in your state.
- Investigate the regulations regarding licensure of the practical nurse in your state.

REVIEW

Briefly answer the following questions.

1. What two steps are necessary to obtain a license for practical nursing?

2. Name two organizations which participate in accreditation programs for practical nursing.

3. State two ways the practical nurse can keep informed on new techniques and policies about nursing.

4. Name two recommended publications for practical nurses.

5. Who is the most important person to consider when working with other team members?

unit 3 personal health and body care

OBJECTIVES

After studying this unit, the student will be able to:

- List four good health habits.
- Give two reasons for good health.
- Name five basics of personal hygiene.
- State the importance of handwashing.
- Explain the need for sleep and rest.

Everyone in the health field must know and practice good health habits and personal hygiene. The practical nurse should be aware of this fact. The nurse is often exposed to infection because of the many contacts with the patients. A healthy body is more resistant to disease. It also promotes mental health. One of the nurse's duties is to teach patients to use correct health practices. Setting the right example is more effective than simply telling him about the importance of personal health and body care.

PERSONAL HYGIENE

The appearance of the nurse affects the morale of the patient. Personal hygiene and clean clothing are essential. A daily bath, use of deodorants, clean underwear, oral hygiene and frequent shampoos are basic to good grooming. A neat appearance helps to gain confidence and respect from patients. Planning helps the nurse to provide time necessary for good grooming.

Personal hygiene also includes thorough and frequent washing of the hands. Handwashing before and after caring for each patient is important in preventing the spread of disease. Soap and running water should be used whenever the hands become contaminated. The fingernails should be kept clean at all times.

Schools of nursing specify rules concerning student health practices. Hospitals set standards of hygiene and conduct to which personnel must conform. All health team

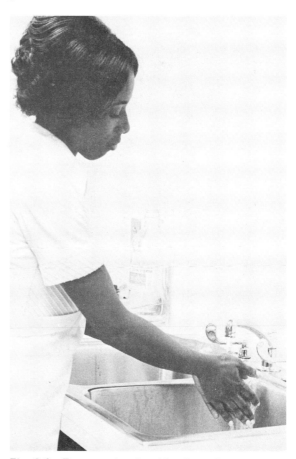

Fig. 3-1 Frequent handwashing is an important aspect of personal hygiene.

personnel must comply with these standards. This is necessary if proper health practices are to be maintained. Nurses should accept this responsibility. They should also urge others to comply.

GOOD HEALTH HABITS

One good health practice is the development of proper food habits. Food supplies energy for the day's activities. Meals should be eaten in a relaxing atmosphere and on a regular schedule. Body weight can more easily be controlled by the amount and kind of food eaten. A balanced diet is essential for the student as well as for the practicing nurse.

Other habits which should be developed are obtaining adequate rest and practicing cor-

rect posture and body mechanics. Rest and sleep requirements vary with the individual. Adequate sleep is necessary to maintain health and prevent undue tension, mental strain and fatigue.

Posture is the relationship of various parts of the body when standing, sitting, lying down, stooping or bending. *Body mechanics* is the way in which the body moves and maintains balance by the most efficient use of its parts. Good posture and the use of correct body mechanics will prevent unnecessary strain and lessen fatigue. The importance of good posture and some basic rules concerning the practice of correct body mechanics are presented later in the text.

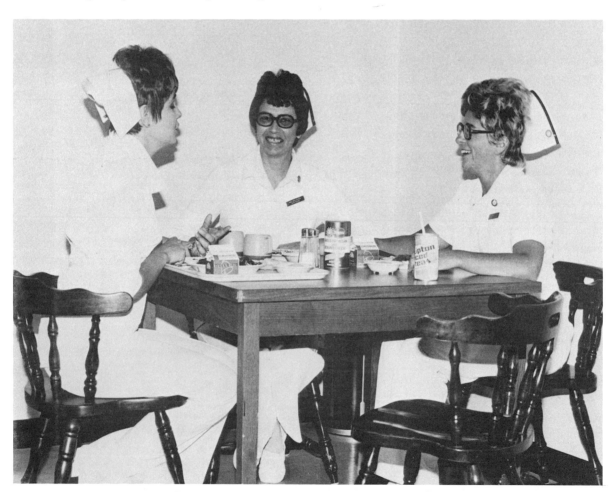

Fig. 3-2 Relaxing over a meal should be part of the day's routine.

VOCABULARY

- Define the following words:

    body mechanics   essential   posture
    compliance   hygiene   resistance
    contamination   morale   standards

SUGGESTED ACTIVITIES

- Visit a local health facility and review the health code established for its employees.

- List and evaluate the health habits and grooming routine you practice daily.

REVIEW

Briefly answer the following questions.

1. Name 4 good health practices.

2. Give 2 reasons for keeping healthy.

3. Name 5 basics which make up good personal hygiene.

4. Why is handwashing important?

5. Give 2 reasons why the body needs sleep and rest.

unit 4 body mechanics and posture

OBJECTIVES

After studying this unit, the student will be able to:

- Define posture and body mechanics.
- Explain the benefits of the practice of good body mechanics.
- List the principles of good body mechanics.

Body mechanics is the way in which the body moves and maintains balance by the most efficient use of all its parts. The nurse is better equipped to give patient care using good body mechanics. Balanced movements reduce fatigue and strain when moving a patient from one position to another. The nurse often cannot depend on help from the patient. Even when assisted by other health team members, the nurse should practice good body mechanics.

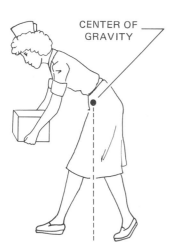

CENTER OF GRAVITY

Posture is the relationship of the various parts of the body when standing, sitting, or lying down. Good posture requires that the body weight be in balance with relation to the spine and the body's center of gravity. The *center of gravity* is the point around which all parts of the body exactly balance each other. Posture determines the distribution of body weight and the pull on the joints and muscles.

Good body alignment for the patient lessens discomfort and induces rest. Proper positioning also promotes good circulation through each body area. This prevents the formation of decubiti (bedsores) caused by prolonged pressure in one area. Muscle contractures are also prevented. A *contracture* is a shortened, inflexible muscle state which results from constant pull on a muscle that is not being used.

The principles of good body mechanics must be applied whenever heavy objects are lifted or carried. The body should be kept in balance at all times. Maximum use of the large, strong muscles will prevent strain on the weaker muscles. The muscles of the hip, thigh, and

When nurses use body mechanics based on sound principles, they protect themselves and the patients from injury.

1. Encourage patients to be as active as is permissible to maintain strength and muscle tone.
2. Maintain a broad base of support by standing with feet comfortably apart. Place one foot forward and point toes in the direction of movement.
3. Flex the knees and hips when stooping, to pick up an object from the floor.
4. Use the longest and strongest muscles of the arms and legs rather than the weaker back muscles.
5. Carry heavy objects close to the body.
6. Move the patient by rolling or turning whenever possible rather than lifting.
7. When turning the patient in bed, roll the patient toward you rather than away from you.

Fig. 4-1 Rules for the practice of good body mechanics

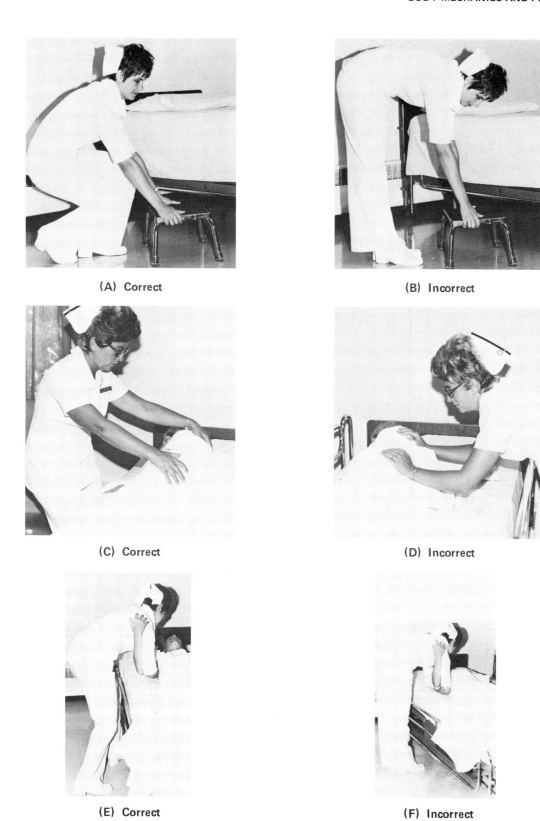

(A) Correct

(B) Incorrect

(C) Correct

(D) Incorrect

(E) Correct

(F) Incorrect

Fig. 4-2 Principles of body mechanics determine which positions are correct.

lower leg are strong and should be used when-every possible. Muscles in the back are weak.

Balance is maintained with the least amount of effort if the center of gravity is over the center of the base of support. The body is more stable (less likely to "topple over") if the center of gravity is low and the base of support is large or broad. The base of support is broadened if the feet are apart.

The center of gravity is lowered by bending the knees instead of bending over from the hips. Facing in the direction of movement and bending the forward knee will help to place the weight on the large thigh muscle and prevent back strain. When carrying heavy objects, the weight is kept nearer the center of gravity if the object is held close to the body.

VOCABULARY

- Define the following words:

alignment	fatigue	stability
balance	mechanics	strain

SUGGESTED ACTIVITIES

- Lift and carry a heavy book using the correct and incorrect positions in figure 4-2. Decide which general area of muscles receives the greatest stress.

- Observe the posture and body alignment of another student while he or she is standing, sitting, and lying down.

REVIEW

A. By circling A or B, indicate which drawing (in each pair) shows the practice of good body mechanics.

1. A   B   2. A   B

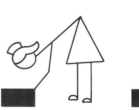 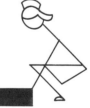

B. Define the following terms.

Posture

Body mechanics

C. Match the definitions in Column I with the correct term in Column II.

	Column I	Column II
_____	1. a shortened, inflexible muscle state	a. strong muscles
_____	2. the point around which all parts of the body balance each other	b. decubiti
_____	3. sores caused by prolonged pressure in one area	c. alignment
_____	4. placing body parts in their proper positions	d. contracture
_____	5. muscles of the hip, thigh, lower leg and arms	e. center of gravity

D. Briefly answer the following questions.

1. List four rules of good body mechanics.

2. Name two benefits the nurse receives by using correct body mechanics.

unit 5 handwashing

OBJECTIVES

After studying this unit, the student will be able to:

- Identify the steps used in good handwashing.
- List the occasions when it is essential to wash the hands.
- State the mechanical and chemical means by which handwashing destroys bacteria.

The simplest way to help prevent the spread of disease is thorough handwashing. Giving bedside care requires constant use of the hands. The nurse should practice good handwashing and take responsibility for reminding others to wash often. Handwashing is necessary:

- Before and after eating
- After using a handkerchief
- After using the toilet
- Before and after any contact with a patient.

Pathogenic (disease-producing) germs can be carried to the mouth, nose, eyes and to food or anything else that the hands can touch. Germs cannot be seen by the naked eye but can be seen under the microscope. Moisture and warmth produce ideal conditions for the growth of bacteria.

MECHANICAL AND CHEMICAL ACTION

Handwashing, done properly, removes bacteria by two means of action, chemical and mechanical. Soap removes bacteria through chemical action. It dissolves the natural oil on the skin and loosens dirt and germs which cling to the oil. Friction brings about the mechanical removal of bacteria. Rubbing soaped hands together or scrubbing them with a brush represents mechanical action.

PROCEDURE

1. Assemble equipment:

   Soap   Paper towels   Hand brush

2. Turn on the water by using a paper towel to handle the faucet.

   Sinks equipped with a foot pedal or faucets with long handles for elbow operation are in common use.

   The faucet is always considered contaminated. The nurse should avoid touching the faucet directly at all times—even after handling contaminated material. It is poor practice to deposit more germs on equipment or fixtures commonly used.

3. Regulate the temperature of the water. Warm water makes more soap lather than cold.

4. Wet both hands holding them downward so that water drains from them carrying bacteria away.

5. Apply liquid soap to the hands if it is available.

   If bar soap must be used, rinse it with water before using it.

6. Work up a lather and rub between the fingers beginning with the tips. Rub the back of each hand with a circular motion.

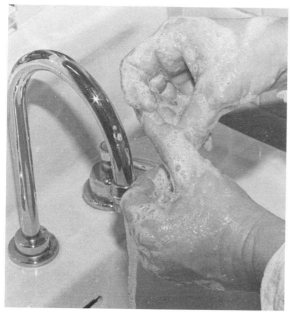

Fig. 5-1 Cleaning under the nails is an important step in handwashing.

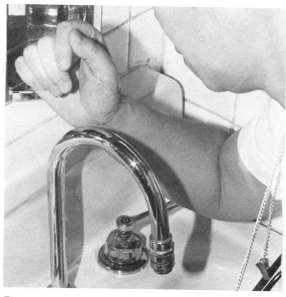

Fig. 5-2 Using the elbow to turn off the faucet prevents soiling freshly washed hands.

7. Clean under each fingernail. Use a brush if necessary.

8. Rinse the hands as they are held downward. Be sure all of the soap is removed.

   Soap residue may cause irritation and chapped skin when left on the hands.

9. Repeat the handwashing for extra cleansing.

10. Use a paper towel to dry both hands. The same paper towel may be used to turn off the faucet.

    Using a towel or the elbow to turn off the faucet prevents recontamination of the hands.

11. Take another towel to finish drying the hands.

    Thorough drying prevents chapping and removes moisture which encourages the growth of bacteria.

VOCABULARY

- Define the following words:

bacteria	friction	pathogenic
chemical	irritation	precaution
contaminated	mechanical	residue

SUGGESTED ACTIVITIES

- Visit a local health care facility and observe the setup of the utility room. Examine and evaluate other areas used for handwashing.

- Discuss other methods used to prevent disease spread such as sterilization and autoclaving.

REVIEW

A. Select the *best* answer.

1. The nurse can best prevent the spread of disease daily by

    a. studying the health code
    b. proper and frequent handwashing
    c. using disposable supplies
    d. checking housekeeping personnel

2. Scrubbing with soap and water is an example of

    a. chemical removal of bacteria
    b. mechanical removal of bacteria
    c. personal hygiene
    d. all of the above

3. Conditions ideal for the growth of pathogenic bacteria are

    a. light and moisture
    b. rough, dry surfaces
    c. darkness and dry surfaces
    d. warmth and moisture

4. Rinsing soap off the hands should be done

    a. with the hands lower than the elbows
    b. so the water drains toward the elbow, rinsing the forearm
    c. rinsing only one hand at a time
    d. so a slight protective residue is left on the skin

5. A paper towel is used to turn off the faucet *after* a thorough hand-washing to

    a. prevent adding more germs to the faucet surface
    b. keep the faucet sterile
    c. prevent recontamination of the hands
    d. keep the hands sterile

B. Briefly answer the following questions.

1. List the occasions when handwashing is essential.

2. List the steps for proper handwashing.

SELF-EVALUATION I

A. Match the items in Column II with the correct definitions in Column I.

Column I

_____ 1. most important part of the practical nurse's duties

_____ 2. disease-producing organisms

_____ 3. ideal conditions for growth of bacteria

_____ 4. an important means of preventing the spread of disease

_____ 5. the way in which the body moves and maintains balance by the most efficient use of all its parts

_____ 6. good diet, sufficient rest, correct posture, and good body mechanics

_____ 7. the oldest practical nursing organization

_____ 8. group of professionally trained persons who use their skills to promote the patient's health

_____ 9. a shortened, inflexible muscle state

_____ 10. housekeeping and food service staff

Column II

a. bedside nursing
b. body mechanics
c. contractures
d. good health habits
e. health team
f. handwashing
g. NAPNES
h. auxiliary workers
i. pathogens
j. warmth and moisture

B. Select the *best* answer.

1. The duties of the practical nurse include
   a. fulfilling assignments carefully and efficiently
   b. respecting religious and cultural beliefs
   c. keeping up with the current trends
   d. all of the above

2. The examinations for practical nurse licensure are made up by the
   a. state board of nursing
   b. NAPNES
   c. National League for Nursing
   d. American Medical Association

3. The code of behavior established by NAPNES relates to
   a. hospital regulations
   b. Public Health Law
   c. ethics
   d. legal restrictions

4. The duties of the health team include

   a. cooperation among staff members
   b. prevention of illness
   c. promotion of health
   d. all of the above

5. The purpose for licensure is to

   a. provide income from license fees
   b. protect the nurse and patient
   c. limit the number of LPNs licensed
   d. none of the above

6. Good body mechanics includes

   a. standing with the feet apart slightly
   b. flexing the knees when stooping
   c. carrying heavy objects close to the body
   d. all of the above

7. The center of gravity is lowered by

   a. bending over from the hips
   b. facing in the direction of movement
   c. flexing the knees
   d. broadening the base of support

8. When turning a patient in bed, the patient should be

   a. rolled away from you   c. lifted whenever possible
   b. rolled toward you   d. none of the above

SECTION II BEDMAKING
unit 6 the closed bed

OBJECTIVES

After studying this unit, the student will be able to:

- Identify the steps used in making a closed bed.
- Explain reasons for completing one side of the bed at a time.
- Explain how to miter a corner.
- Describe the way to insert a pillow in the pillowcase.

Since most hospitals use a standard size bed, bedmaking procedures do not vary greatly. Generally the patient's bed is twenty-six inches high; this height is convenient for giving bedside care. The head of the bed can be raised and the foot of the bed lowered. This is done by turning a crank or pushing an electrical control button. Electric controls can be easily operated by the patient.

MAKING THE CLOSED BED

A closed bed is an unassigned, unoccupied bed. The closed bed is made after a patient has been discharged or just before a new patient is admitted. The bed and entire unit which had been occupied by the patient must be thoroughly cleaned before the closed bed is made. The bed then remains closed until a new patient is admitted. Bedrest may be a major part of the patient's treatment. The patient who spends many days or weeks in the hospital should have comfort and rest provided by a well-made bed.

PROCEDURE

1. Assemble equipment — arrange in order of use:

   2 pillowcases
   Spread
   Blanket
   2 large sheets (90" by 108")
   Drawsheet
   Plastic or rubber drawsheet*
   Mattress pad and/or cover

   * Hospital mattresses which are treated with plastic do not require the protection of a moisture-proof sheet.

2. Lock the wheels of the bed and place a chair at the side of the bed.

3. Arrange linen on the chair so the first item needed is on top.

   Organizing the linen needed for bedmaking saves steps. Learn to make the most efficient use of time and energy.

4. Fit the mattress cover over the mattress and adjust the corners smoothly.

   Work entirely from one side of the bed until that side is completed.

5. If a mattress pad is used, place it even with the top of the mattress and unfold.

   Smooth out all wrinkles in the pad.

6. Place and unfold the bottom sheet right side up, wide hem at the top. The small hem should be brought to the foot of the mattress.

   Center fold should be at the center of the bed. Avoid "shaking out" the sheet since this spreads germs around the room. Unfold the sheet slowly. The bottom end of the mattress is not covered.

7. Tuck the bottom sheet under the top of the mattress and make a mitered corner, figure 6-1.

   Sheet should be long enough to fold 12 to 18 inches under the mattress.

8. Tuck in the sheet on one side. Work from the head to the foot of the bed.

   To keep the sheet straight on the bed, use the center fold as a guide.

9. If the mattress is not moisture proof, lay a protective drawsheet across the center of the mattress.

10. Place a cotton drawsheet directly over the protective drawsheet; completely cover it. Tuck both drawsheets under the mattress together. Begin in the center and work toward the head of the bed. Then finish tucking in from center toward the foot of the bed.

    Working from the center prevents the drawsheet from becoming crooked and wrinkled. The cotton drawsheet should extend at least 2" above and below the protective drawsheet to prevent the plastic or rubber from touching the patient's skin.

11. Place the top sheet, wrong side up with stitching of the hem showing. The hem should be even with the upper edge of the mattress.

12. Place the blanket on the bed with the top edge about 8" below head of mattress.

13. Place spread with top hem even with head of mattress. Unfold spread to the foot of the bed.

14. Tuck the top sheet, blanket and spread under the mattress at the foot of the bed and make a mitered corner.

When one side of the bed is complete, the other side can be finished easily.

15. Go to the other side of the bed and continue with the procedure.

16. Fanfold the top covers to the center of the bed in order to work with the bottom sheet and pad.

17. Tuck the bottom sheet under the head of the mattress and make a mitered corner.

    Working from top to bottom, smooth out all wrinkles and tighten the sheet as much as possible. Wrinkles can cause the patient discomfort and may lead to the formation of bedsores.

18. Continue to tuck in the drawsheets, top sheet, blanket and spread as was done on the opposite side.

19. Fold top sheet back over blanket, making 8-inch cuff.

    This protects the patient's skin from the coarseness of the blanket.

20. Insert the pillow into its case:

    a. Use one hand inside the pillowcase to separate the sides and free the corners.

       The sides of freshly laundered and pressed cases often stick together.

    b. Grasp the end seam of the pillowcase from the outside. Turn the case back over the hand.

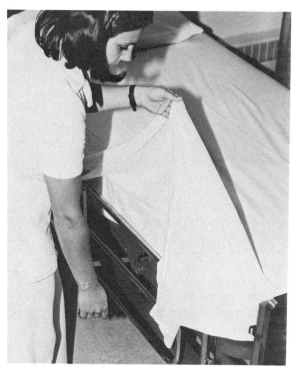

(A) Lift the hanging sheet about 12 inches from the end of the bed.

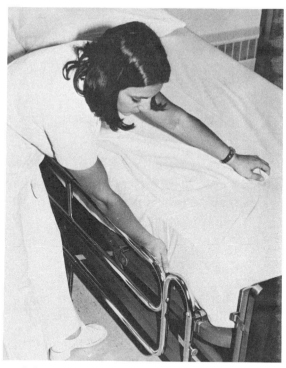

(B) Tuck the lower portion under the mattress.

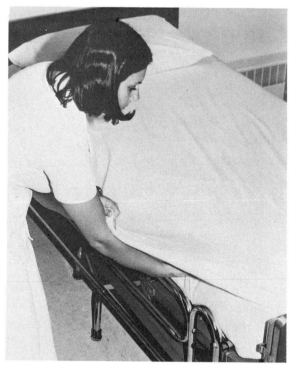

(C) Hold the fold with one hand. Bring the triangle down.

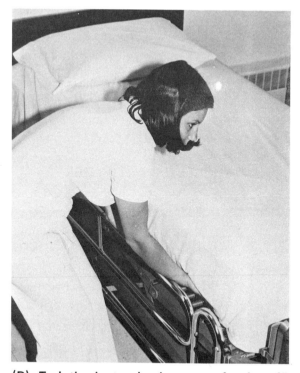

(D) Tuck the sheet under the mattress forming a 45 degree angle.

Fig. 6-1 Making a mitered corner (A-D)

c. Release the hand grip under the case just enough to grasp the pillow.

d. With the other hand, fit the pillow into the corners of the case.

e. Pull the case over the entire length of the pillow.

Make a lengthwise pleat in pillowcase if necessary to provide better fit. Place fold on underside of pillow facing foot of bed.

21. Place the pillow at the head of the bed.

Check to see that the open end of pillowcase is away from the door.

22. Pull the spread to the head of the bed so it fits smoothly over the pillow.

23. Return the overbed table and chair to the original position.

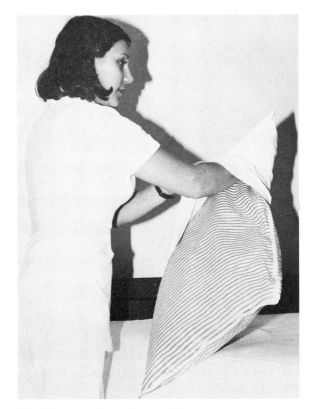

Fig. 6-2 Both the pillow and the case are held away from the uniform.

VOCABULARY

- Define the following words:

convenient	lengthwise	pleat
drawsheet	miter	wrinkle
fanfold		

SUGGESTED ACTIVITIES

- Collect the linen needed to make a closed bed. Use whatever kind of bed is available and prepare to make the bed using the procedure described in this unit. Obtain a clock or watch and keep a record of the time needed to make a closed bed correctly.

- Strip the bed, refold the linen and begin again to remake the bed. This time, keeping a record of the minutes, make the bed alternating often between sides of the bed and taking linen from a disorderly stack. Compare the two times and the quality of the bedmaking.

- Demonstrate how to insert a pillow into a pillowcase.

REVIEW

Briefly answer the following questions.

1. When is a closed bed made?

2. What benefits come from making one side of the bed at a time?

3. Why are the sheets unfolded rather than shaken out?

4. Why is it important to pull the bottom sheet tight leaving no wrinkles?

5. Making a cuff by folding the top sheet back over the blanket performs what function?

6. Name four steps used to make a mitered corner.

7. Describe the proper way to insert a pillow in a pillowcase.

unit 7 opening the bed

OBJECTIVES

After studying this unit, the student will be able to:

- List the steps taken to open a closed bed.
- Explain the meaning an open bed has to the patient.
- Describe how to fanfold the bedcovers.

The open bed is a welcome sign to the patient. It indicates that the patient's arrival has been expected and that the health team is ready to give him care. The bed is opened by fanfolding the top bedcovers to the end of the bed or to the halfway point. This detail will vary in different health facilities. The bed should not be opened until shortly before the patient's arrival. If the bed lies open for a long time before occupancy, dust and germs in the air will settle on the sheets and pillowcase.

PROCEDURE

1. Working at the bedside, fold the top edge of the spread over the edge of the blanket if there is one. (Some hospital beds are made up with sheets and a bedspread.)
2. Fold the sheet down over the blanket and spread.
3. Face the foot of the bed. Grasp the upper edges of the top bedding with both hands.

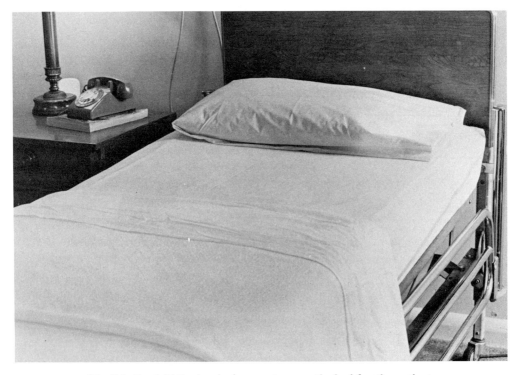

Fig. 7-1 Fanfold the top bedcovers to open the bed for the patient.

Hands should be well separated. This gives a wide grasp on the covers and makes for easier control and handling.

4. Fanfold the covers down to the middle or foot of the bed, figure 7-1.

Fold should be the same width as the top fold. The top sheet fold must constantly remain on top of the fold.

5. Check the bottom sheet for wrinkles; retighten the sheet if necessary.

VOCABULARY

- Define the following words.

manipulation
fanfold

grasp
significance

SUGGESTED ACTIVITIES

- Make a closed bed and practice fanfolding the top spread and sheet.
- Compare the bedmaking procedures of local hospitals and nursing homes.

REVIEW

Briefly answer the following questions.

1. How far are the bedcovers folded?

2. Where should the nurse stand to fanfold the top covers?

3. What meaning does an open bed have for a patient?

4. State the disadvantage of opening the bed too far ahead of the patient's arrival.

5. List the steps for opening the bed.

unit 8 the occupied bed

OBJECTIVES

After studying this unit, the student will be able to:

- Describe how to change the linen on an occupied bed.

- Explain how to get the patient's cooperation.

Unless the patient is permitted out of bed by the doctor's order, his bed is made while he is in it. The patient frequently enjoys this refreshing procedure if the nurse is skillful. Making the bed usually follows the bed bath.

In order to perform all necessary routines and to give priority to those procedures which must be performed at a given time, keeping a schedule is essential. It is suggested, therefore, that the practical nurse avoid using the expression, "Would you like to have your bed made now?". It is better to say, "I am ready to make your bed now." The nurse will discover other expressions that aid in gaining the patient's cooperation. Before performing this procedure, the nurse should understand correct ways of moving and turning the patient in bed.

PROCEDURE

1. Assemble the equipment:

   Cotton drawsheet
   2 large sheets
   2 pillowcases

2. Greet the patient and explain the procedure.

   Address the patient by name or check the ID arm bracelet. Explaining the procedure helps relieve anxiety and gain cooperation from the patient.

3. Arrange the bed and the linen.

   a. Place bedside chair at the foot of the bed.

   b. Arrange linen on the chair in order of use; the first item would be a clean sheet (for bottom); then drawsheet, sheet, spread, pillowcases.

   c. Screen the unit.

   The patient's need for privacy should be respected.

   d. Lock the wheels. Adjust the bed so that the head and foot are flat.

   The bed should be flat during bedmaking unless the patient's condition does not permit it.

4. Loosen the bedding from beneath the mattress on all sides.

   Lift edge of mattress with one hand and draw bedding out with the other. This prevents tearing the sheets and avoids jarring the patient.

5. Except for the sheet, remove top covers (spread and blanket) one at a time; fold each toward the bottom of the bed, pick it up in the center, and place over the back of the chair.

6. Lay a clean sheet over the soiled top sheet. Have the patient hold on to the top of the clean sheet while you pull out the soiled one.

Do not expose the patient more than is required.

7. Help the patient turn to the side of the bed toward the nurse. Raise the siderail. Support the patient with a pillow. The patient may grasp the siderail for extra support.

Protect the patient from falling out of bed. Do not proceed until the patient is comfortable and safe.

8. Go to the other side of the bed and prepare to change the bottom sheet and the drawsheet.

9. Loosen the soiled bottom sheet and roll it lengthwise to the center of the bed. Roll the drawsheet in the same manner.

Place sheets as close to the patient as possible. This makes it easier to pull them through the other side.

10. Place the clean bottom sheet lengthwise on the bed. The narrow hem should come to the edge of the mattress at the foot; the lengthwise center fold of the sheet should be at the center of the bed.

The smooth side of the hem should face the patient.

11. Tuck in the top of the sheet at the head of the bed; miter the corner.

12. Tuck in the sheet along the side of the bed.

Working toward the foot of the bed keeps the sheet properly centered.

13. Pull the protective drawsheet back into place. Lay the cotton drawsheet over the protective drawsheet.

The cotton drawsheet must completely cover the protective drawsheet. Be sure the sheets are tight and free of wrinkles.

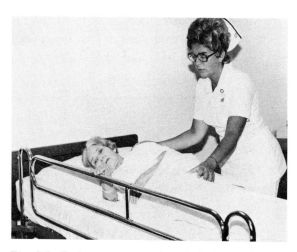

Fig. 8-1 Patients can sometimes help by holding on the siderail.

14. Fanfold the bottom sheet and the two drawsheets as close to the patient's back as possible.

Be sure the soiled sheets and the clean sheets are not tangled in the center of the bed. Fanfold the clean bottom sheet over the soiled sheet.

15. Help the patient to turn toward you. Raise the siderail. Support the patient with a pillow.

Allow the patient to rest if the bed-making procedure becomes tiring. A weak patient may easily become fatigued.

16. Go to the other side of the bed. Prepare to remove the soiled linen which has been gathered behind the patient.

17. Lower the rail on the side opposite the patient.

18. Ask the patient to hold the siderail he is facing.

Gently pull the soiled linen away to prevent jarring the patient or injuring his skin.

19. Fold the soiled linen loosely and place in the hamper.

Keep soiled linen away from the uniform. Avoid shaking the linen while removing it.

20. Pull the bottom sheet and the drawsheet tight; tuck them both in.

21. Help the patient to a comfortable position. Replace the pillow. Straighten out the top sheet.

22. Replace the blanket and spread. Tuck them in at the foot of the bed together with the top sheet.

Make a toe pleat in the top covers for the patient's comfort.

23. Place the signal cord within the patient's reach.

24. Replace bedside table and chair.

25. Remove soiled linens and leave unit in neat condition.

VOCABULARY

- Define the following words:

alert	jarring	rational
conserve	postpone	routine
expose	privacy	schedule
flexible	refreshing	self-worth

SUGGESTED ACTIVITIES

- Role play the following problem situations. After the situation has been presented, evaluate the nurse's tact and efficiency in caring for the patient.
  a. An older woman is enjoying reading a book. She does not want to be disturbed to have her bed made. Her physician has not yet permitted her to get out of bed. How may the nurse gain her cooperation?
  b. An adolescent boy who has been brought up by his father alone is uncomfortable and embarrassed when the nurse begins to make his bed. How can she make him feel at ease?

- Make an occupied bed using the procedure described in the unit. Ask another student to lie in the bed while you change the linen.

REVIEW

Select the *best* answer.

1. Making the occupied bed is necessary when the patient
   a. has visitors
   b. wants extra attention
   c. is up and about
   d. is not permitted out of bed

2. Before making the occupied bed, the nurse should review the correct way to
   a. move and turn the patient in bed
   b. clean floor and wall surfaces
   c. clean equipment in the patient's unit
   d. fold clean bed linens

3. Making an occupied bed usually follows

   a. making an unoccupied bed   c. serving lunch
   b. taking a rectal temperature   d. giving a bed bath

4. A kind but firm way to approach the patient when preparing to change the bed linen is to say

   a. "Are you ready to have me make your bed?"
   b. "How about getting ready for your linen change?"
   c. "I am ready to make your bed now."
   d. "I'm ready when you are."

5. The position of the bed during bedmaking is

   a. flat at all times
   b. with the foot of the bed raised
   c. with the head of the bed raised
   d. flat, if the patient's condition permits

6. The clean top sheet

   a. covers the patient through most of the bedmaking
   b. is the last sheet to be placed against the patient
   c. is rolled under the soiled sheet
   d. is fanfolded lengthwise

7. To assist the patient to turn in bed

   a. push the patient to the opposite side of the bed
   b. pull the patient toward you
   c. assure him that siderails are not needed
   d. place a pillow under his head

8. To position the cotton drawsheet and the protective drawsheet

   a. leave a fold in the cotton drawsheet
   b. roll the cotton drawsheet under the protective drawsheet
   c. cover the protective drawsheet completely with the cotton drawsheet
   d. tuck them both in at the head of the bed

9. The soiled linen should be removed from the bed

   a. with one fast pull
   b. with a gentle shake
   c. by gently pulling it
   d. while turning the patient on his back

10. The top bedding is made comfortable for the patient by

   a. letting them hang loosely at the end of the bed
   b. making a toe pleat in the covers
   c. tucking the covers in tightly around the end corners
   d. leaving the spread off most of the time

unit 9 the postoperative bed

OBJECTIVES

After studying this unit, the student will be able to:

- Name ways the postoperative bed benefits the patient.
- List the special features of beds used in the recovery room.
- Describe the steps used in making a postoperative bed.

Following surgery, patients are usually transferred to the recovery room. Many hospitals use the postoperative bed only within that area. However, the procedure for making a postoperative bed in the patient's unit is the same as in the recovery room.

BENEFITS TO THE PATIENT

The nurse prepares the postoperative bed after the patient has been taken to surgery. The postoperative bed is made so the patient is disturbed as little as possible while the linens are changed. The sheets are folded in a way which permits an easy and quick transfer of the patient to the bed, figure 9-1. After surgery, the patient is usually weak and not alert; this postoperative bed helps the patient by making the transfer simpler.

BEDS WITH SPECIALIZED FEATURES

In health facilities having a recovery room or intensive care unit, a special bed is

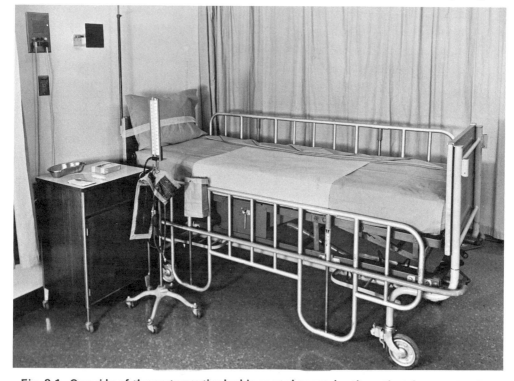

Fig. 9-1 One side of the postoperative bed is opened to receive the patient from a stretcher.

used, figure 9-2. The patient is transferred to this bed from the operating table and is taken to the specialized care area. The patient is transferred back to his own unit in the same bed. Features of the bed that simplify the care of the patient after surgery are:

- The head and footboards are removable.

- The bed is narrower than the regular hospital bed. This allows for easy passage through doors and corridors of the hospital.

- Overhead or lateral fracture equipment may be mounted on the bed.

- The intravenous (I.V.) pole may be used in six different locations: two at the head of the bed, two at the foot of the bed, and two at the center section of the bed.

The pole is specially designed so that solution bottles hang securely in place.

PROCEDURE

1. Assemble equipment and articles needed by a postoperative patient:

   I.V. pole
   Paper bag and safety pins
   Protective drawsheet
   Cotton drawsheet
   Tongue depressor
   Emesis basin

2. Lock the wheels of the bed and lower the siderails.

3. Tuck the bottom sheet in according to the instructions for making a closed bed.

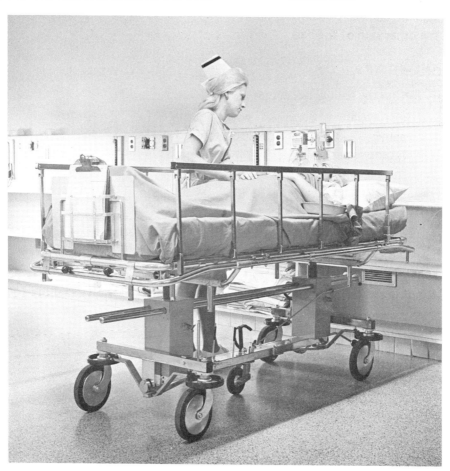

Fig. 9-2 Beds used in the recovery room are designed for safety and easy access to the patient.

4. Place a protective drawsheet and a cotton drawsheet across the *head* of the bed. Miter the corners. Tuck in the two drawsheets on both sides. Be sure the protective drawsheet is completely covered.

   This protects the mattress and provides for easy linen change.

5. Place the top sheet, blanket and spread over the end of the bed without tucking them in.

6. Fold the top bedding back toward the head of the bed. This should leave the edge of the bedding even with the edge of the mattress.

7. Fanfold the top bedding to the side of the bed.

   The patient can be transferred easily into the other side of the bed.

8. Place the pillow upright at the head of the bed.

   The patient's head should lie flat after surgery. The pillow remaining upright protects the patient's head if restlessness should occur.

9. Place only those articles needed on the bedside stand.

10. Pin a paper bag to the siderail near the head of the bed.

    This will be used for discard of gauze or paper tissues.

11. Clear a path for the stretcher or bed which is occupied by the patient.

    Be alert to assist health team members as the patient is returned to the room. Raise the siderails as soon as the patient is placed in the bed.

VOCABULARY

- Define the following words:

disturbed	postoperative	specialized
gauze	recovery room	stretcher
intensive care unit	restlessness	surgery
intravenous		

SUGGESTED ACTIVITIES

- Inspect the type of bed which is used in the recovery room or the intensive care unit. Look for the special features identified earlier in this unit.
- Gather the necessary sheets, covers, and pillow. Practice making a postoperative bed. Use the method explained in this unit. Check each step of the procedure.

REVIEW

Briefly answer the following questions.

1. When is the postoperative bed prepared?

2. Name two ways in which placement of the top bedding in the post-operative bed differs from that of the open bed.

3. Name three special features of the beds which are used in the recovery room.

4. Give two reasons why the postoperative bed is made.

SELF-EVALUATION II

Select the *best* answer.

1. The drawsheet should be tucked in over the head of the bed, when making a(an)

   a. open bed
   b. occupied bed
   c. closed bed
   d. postoperative bed

2. To prevent the protective drawsheet from touching the patient's skin, the cotton drawsheet should

   a. be of the same size
   b. extend the full length of the bed
   c. completely cover the protective drawsheet
   d. be smooth

3. A bed height convenient for giving bedside care is

   a. 13 inches
   b. 32 inches
   c. 26 inches
   d. 8 inches

4. Wrinkles in the bottom sheet can cause

   a. discomfort
   b. decubiti
   c. restlessness
   d. all of the above

5. The best way to gain the patient's cooperation in bedmaking is to say

   a. "Are you ready to have me make your bed?"
   b. "How about getting ready for your linen change?"
   c. "I am ready to make your bed now."
   d. "I'm ready when you are."

6. The postoperative bed is prepared

   a. after the patient has been taken to surgery
   b. in order to make transfer of the patient to the bed easier
   c. in order to change the bed linen without disturbing the patient too much
   d. all of the above

7. A bed in the recovery room

   a. has a removable head and footboard
   b. is extra wide to hold needed equipment for the patient
   c. has only one attachment for the I.V. bottles
   d. has padded rails on all sides to protect the patient

8. A pillow is placed upright at the head of the postoperative bed to

   a. keep drafts away from the patient's head
   b. protect the patient's head if he is restless and moves about
   c. prevent staining the head of the bed
   d. keep it handy for later use

9. The nurse should complete one side of the bed before going to the other side in order to

   a. keep an eye on the patient
   b. straighten the top covers together
   c. prevent wasting time and effort with unnecessary movement
   d. make the toe pleat at the right time

10. The purpose of forming the toe pleat when making an occupied bed is to

    a. make room for the patient's feet
    b. make the bed more attractive
    c. better prepare the patient for surgery
    d. convert a closed bed into an open bed

SECTION III THE PATIENT'S HOSPITAL ENVIRONMENT

unit 10 care and use of room equipment

OBJECTIVES

After studying this unit, the student will be able to:

- Identify the uses of specific pieces of standard equipment found in the hospital unit.

- Explain the importance of order and cleanliness.

- Describe the ideal environmental conditions of a hospital unit.

Environment affects the health and comfort of the patient both physically and mentally. A cheerful, pleasant room helps give the patient a sense of well-being and recovery. A depressing or uncomfortable setting increases anxiety and tension, two major handicaps to recovery from illness.

STANDARD EQUIPMENT

The patient unit usually consists of a hospital bed with or without siderails, bedside cabinet, overbed table, chair, and overbed light. Furniture and equipment will vary depending on three factors:

a. type of room (ward, semiprivate or private)

b. type of medical service provided for that patient

c. the specific needs of the patient

The Overbed Table

The overbed table is a standard piece of equipment in most patient units. The table can be moved around the room easily and can be adjusted for different heights. These two factors give the overbed table many uses. The

nurse may need to adjust it for each particular use. Whether the patient is reading, writing, or eating, the height of the table should be comfortable and not cause strain.

For a patient who has dyspnea or orthopnea, use of the overbed table may assist breathing. *Dyspnea* is a condition in which the patient has difficulty breathing. *Orthopnea* is a respiratory condition which makes breathing difficult unless the patient is in an upright position. Leaning forward with

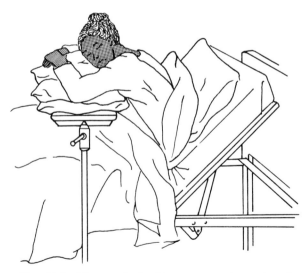

Fig. 10-1 The overbed table supports the patient in the orthopneic position.

arms and head resting on a pillow placed on the overbed table provides rest and an easier breathing position. When the table is used for this purpose, the head of the bed is raised. Pillows are placed at the patient's back and shoulders.

Siderails

Siderails, also called bedrails, act as a safety measure to prevent a patient from falling out of bed. Siderails are attached to modern hospital beds. They extend either the full length of the bed or two-thirds of the length from the head of the bed. On older hospital beds, siderails attach separately. The nurse should be careful to see that the rails are applied securely.

Policies of some health facilities require that patients be protected by raising the siderails at night. A written request by the patient is needed to have the rails remain down. The nurse can be held responsible for injuries a patient receives if the fall occurs as the result of neglect. As a rule, patients who especially need the safety of siderails are those who are: restless, aged, anesthetized, heavily sedated, and/or irrational.

Restraints as well as siderails may be required to confine a patient to the bed. Note: Restraints can never be applied without a doctor's order. Legal action can be taken by the patient or the family if a nurse applies restraints without permission. The only time restraints may be applied without an order is for emergencies. The decision would be made by the nurse in charge. Restraints and siderails exist for the patient's protection; they are not to be used for staff convenience.

IMPORTANCE OF ORDER AND CLEANLINESS

Cleanliness and order are important to the appearance of the unit and the upkeep of the equipment. The nurse should correct and/or report any sign of improper cleaning methods. Cleanliness is important to health maintenance, but it also affects the attitude of the patient. Careless cleaning of the unit may depress or irritate the patient.

Order is usually appreciated by both the patient and the nurse. Health team members show concern when they carefully place furniture and special equipment. Only equipment and supplies which are used in giving the patient proper care should be in the unit. Unnecessary items should be removed or disposed of. Patients sharing a room should keep their supplies and furniture near their beds. One patient's unit should not be used as a temporary storage place for another patient's belongings.

Equipment brought into a room should be clean and orderly. If a tray is used, instruments or equipment should be laid out neatly and covered with a clean towel or paper. Good handwashing should precede the handling of tray items.

Patients often bring personal items with them to the hospital. They may also receive gifts while they are in the hospital. Such items should be placed so they do not disturb the order of the unit. However, since patients enjoy the presence of familiar things, these items should also be within reach.

MAINTAINING THE PROPER ENVIRONMENT

The patient has no way of controlling the heat, lighting or ventilation of his unit. The nurse must adjust these factors for the patient's comfort. When there are two or more persons in the same room, the nurse should not make adjustments for one patient if it is not desired by the group.

Ventilation

Ventilation means allowing fresh air to circulate throughout a room so that stagnant air

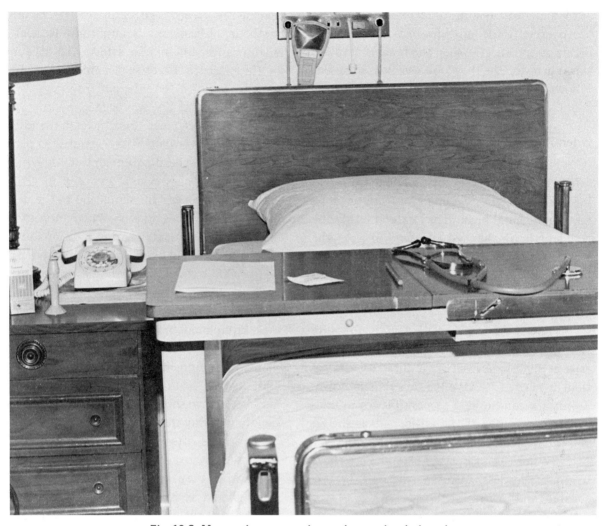

Fig. 10-2 Most patients appreciate a clean and orderly unit.

may be replaced. Natural ventilation is provided by opening windows and doors. Opening windows from the top and the bottom provides for the movement of air. Warm air will rise and go out the upper opening; cool air will enter through the lower opening.

The presence of odors in a hospital ward is disturbing to patients. The nurse should search for the source of bad odors and try to eliminate them. If managed properly, ventilation helps to remove odors.

Temperature

The temperature of the room also affects the patient's comfort and health. Enough heat should be provided so that even in winter some ventilation is possible. Certain medical conditions require different room temperatures and humidity. However, the nurse should know the acceptable standard. Rooms should be about 70°F (21°C), especially if there are several patients in a ward. Individual adjustments may be made by varying the number of bedcovers. In a private room the temperature may be regulated as the patient wishes.

Lighting

Patient units usually have a central overhead light, and an overbed light which may be used for reading or for providing visibility during the night. However, overbed lights which remain on throughout the night often make it difficult for patients to sleep. Although some light is necessary, the nurse should consider the patient's need for sleep. Many hospitals have small nightlights along the base of the walls; these make nursing care possible with a minimum of disturbance. In those units where these nightlights are not in use, turning on a nearby light (e.g. bathroom) or using a flashlight is sufficient.

Noise

Of all environmental conditions, excess noise probably produces the most tension. Hospital designers try to eliminate noise through the use of soundproofing. In spite of this, noise in the hall may be heard in many rooms. The nurse can reduce the noise level by placing door silencers where needed, and seeing that movable equipment is well oiled. The nurse should try to develop a quiet manner and a soft but clear voice. All hospital personnel need to be aware of the importance of quiet.

VOCABULARY

- Define the following words:

accessible	elevated	orthopnea
anesthesia	emergency	permission
anxiety	environment	restraints
appreciate	erect	sedated
circulate	handicaps	soundproofing
contribute	irrational	tension
depressing	negligence	ventilation
dyspnea		

SUGGESTED ACTIVITIES

- Obtain permission to review the policies of a local health facility. Study policies on siderails and the use of restraints. Report your findings to the class for discussion.

- Ask another student to sit in a hospital bed which has the head elevated. Use pillows and the overbed table to assist the student into an orthopneic position.

REVIEW

Briefly answer the following questions.

1. Name three factors which influence the choice of equipment and furniture for a patient's room.

2. List five standard pieces of furniture or equipment usually found in a patient unit. .

3. What is the purpose of assisting a patient into orthopneic position?

4. What two advantages does the overbed table have which make it especially useful in patient care?

5. What is the purpose of raising the siderails on a patient's bed?

6. Name five patient conditions which definitely require the siderails to be raised.

7. When can restraints be applied without a doctor's written order?

8. Where in the room should the patient's personal items be placed?

9. Name four factors, in the room environment, which may affect the patient's comfort and recovery.

10. Give two reasons for keeping the patient's room clean and orderly.

unit 11 cleaning the room or unit

OBJECTIVES

After studying this unit, the student will be able to:

- Identify methods for cleaning equipment and supplies.
- Explain how to prepare equipment for central supply.
- Explain the steps used to clean a unit.

Daily cleaning of the patient's room (or small separate unit) is called *concurrent cleaning*. This consists of keeping the room neat and orderly, damp mopping the floors, and dusting with a damp cloth. Cleaning that is done after the patient is discharged or moved to another unit is called *terminal cleaning*. The housekeeping department usually provides this service. However, proper destruction and disposal of used supplies, cleaning and replacement of equipment, and thorough cleaning of the area occupied by the patient should be checked by the nurse. Prevention of disease is a major objective of nursing care. Elimination of airborne germs helps prevent the spread of disease. Everything in the room or unit must be kept clean during the patient's stay in the hospital and upon discharge. This includes equipment as well as the area occupied by the patient.

EQUIPMENT AND SUPPLIES

Equipment requires careful handling. Breakage can easily occur if the nurse becomes careless while cleaning the equipment. Hidden cracks or broken wires may cause injuries. Waiting for equipment to be replaced may also delay the care needed by a patient. Any difficulty in handling or operating equipment should be reported. The nurse should ask for instruction and/or assistance before handling unfamiliar equipment.

Nondisposable equipment and supplies need to be washed and rinsed, then sent to central supply department to be sterilized. The functions of the central supply department usually include repair, cleaning, sterilizing, packaging, and distribution of equipment. Contaminated items are cleaned and sterilized by trained personnel according to standardized procedures. This practice has resulted in reducing infections. Smaller hospitals may not have a central supply department. In these facilities, the nurse may be responsible for cleaning the equipment.

PROCEDURE

1. Remove all nondisposable equipment from the bedside stand and take it to the utility room.

2. Rinse equipment soiled with blood or body secretions in cool, running water.

   Hot water causes these substances to coagulate, changing them to a semisolid mass. This makes removal more difficult.

3. Clean thoroughly with hot, soapy water. Remove as many stains as possible.

4. Remove all soap by rinsing well.

5. Dry completely.

   This prevents metal instruments from rusting.

6. After cleaning the equipment, send it to central supply to be sterilized.

Facilities which cannot autoclave or sterilize equipment require health personnel to soak the equipment in 5% creosol solution for 20 minutes.

Disposable equipment is widely used because it reduces the risk of spreading germs. Nondisposable equipment frequently transfers germs because of improper cleaning. Most disposable items are used only once and then discarded.

CLEANING THE UNIT

To clean a unit properly, the use of soap, water, and friction is needed. In addition, the unit should be exposed to fresh air and sunshine. Each of these methods helps to remove bacteria and dust particles. Many bacteria can cause disease; dust irritates the mucous membranes when inhaled. The following procedure describes how to clean the unit.

PROCEDURE

1. Assemble the necessary materials:

   Basin of warm water
   Brown soap or soap powder
   Brush
   2 cleaning cloths
   Laundry bag
   Newspaper for waste
   Scouring powder
   Stretcher

2. Any special equipment used by the patient, such as suction apparatus and oxygen equipment, should be cleaned according to hospital policy and removed from the unit.

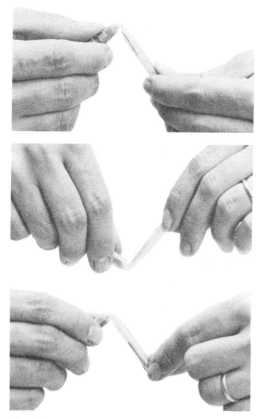 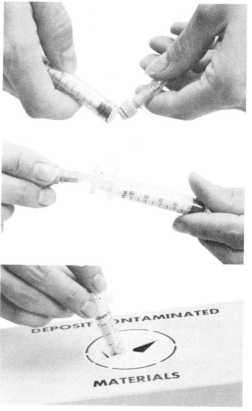

Fig. 11-1 Proper destruction and disposal of used equipment (such as disposable syringes) will help reduce the spread of infection.

Hospital policies differ on the procedure for cleaning special equipment.

3. Remove all disposable materials and personal items such as a toothbrush and leftover face cream. Wrap these in a newspaper to be burned.

   NOTE: Do not discard anything which may be claimed by the patient or by members of his family.

4. Strip the bed and deposit the linen in a laundry hamper. Place the pillows on a chair.

   Blankets when soiled should also be sent to the laundry, or sterilized in some other manner.

5. Take the plastic drawsheet to the utility room and wash it with soap and water. Rinse and dry it thoroughly.

   When possible, hang the plastic drawsheet over a rod to dry and use another one when remaking the bed.

6. Move a stretcher parallel to the bed. With assistance, slide the mattress from the bed to the stretcher.

7. Place the uncovered pillows on the mattress.

8.. Dry dust the coils of the bedsprings, using a long-handled brush.

9. Use one cleaning cloth for washing and one for drying. Proceed as follows:

   a. Wash the framework of the bed, including bedsprings.

   b. Wash the bedside stand inside and out. Leave drawers open to air.

   c. Wash the chair.

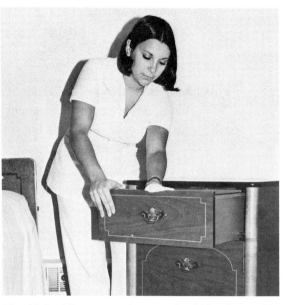

Fig. 11-2 All room equipment should be thoroughly washed after the patient has been discharged or transferred.

Remove stains with scouring powder or detergent. Dry thoroughly to prevent rusting. Change water frequently if it becomes soapy and dirty.

10. Wring out one cloth in clear water without soap. Damp dust surfaces of mattress and pillows.

    Avoid soaking the mattress and pillows.

11. Air the bed as long as possible to be sure all moisture has evaporated. Replace the mattress with assistance.

12. Make a closed bed and leave the unit in order.

    Place the bedside stand on the left side near head of bed. Leave the overbed table across the bottom of the bed. Place chair near the foot of the bed.

VOCABULARY

- Define the following words:

autoclave	coagulate	defective
breakage	creosol	exposed

45

mucous membrane   semisolid   transmit
secretions   sterilized

SUGGESTED ACTIVITIES

- Ask the instructor to arrange a tour through a central supply department. Observe the placement of soiled and clean articles. Examine machines used for sterilizing supplies.

- If possible, seek out a health worker or employee who has worked in central supply for a few years. Briefly discuss the kinds of supplies which have been replaced by the use of disposable items.

REVIEW

Match the statements in column I with the correct term in column II.

Column I	Column II
_____ 1. solution used for sterilizing equipment	a. dust
_____ 2. used with soap and water	b. central supply
_____ 3. irritates the mucous membranes	c. creosol
_____ 4. department where supplies are sterilized	d. housekeeping
_____ 5. supplies which reduce the spread of germs	e. friction
_____ 6. usually cleans rooms and/or units	f. bedside stand
_____ 7. usually placed at the left side of the bed	g. disposable items
_____ 8. prevents coagulation of body secretions on metal surfaces	h. cold water

SELF-EVALUATION III

A. Select the *best* answer.

1. Environment affects the health and comfort of the patient
   - a. physically but not mentally
   - b. mentally but not physically
   - c. physically and mentally
   - d. only slightly

2. The overbed table
   - a. is helpful to the patient with orthopnea
   - b. does not need height adjustments
   - c. should be used only for meals
   - d. should remain near the foot of the bed

3. Siderails of the bed should be raised
   - a. if the patient is heavily sedated
   - b. only if the doctor writes an order
   - c. only when the patient requests it
   - d. if the patient is over 65

4. Proper ventilation of a room
   - a. is provided by opening the door slightly
   - b. requires an electrical appliance
   - c. automatically humidifies the room
   - d. requires two openings for the movement of air

5. Excessive noise must be avoided because
   - a. patients cannot hear the television programs
   - b. nurses find it unpleasant
   - c. it produces tension
   - d. it interferes with giving care

6. The well-being of the patient is helped by
   - a. a bright overbed light during night rounds
   - b. communicating in a loud voice
   - c. a room temperature of 74°F or 23°C
   - d. proper ventilation of the room

7. The standard temperature for the hospital room is
   - a. 63°F or 17°C
   - b. 74°F or 23°C
   - c. 70°F or 21°C
   - d. 77°F or 25°C

8. Tension may occur as the result of
   - a. loud noises
   - b. glaring lights
   - c. unpleasant odors
   - d. all of the above

9. Instruments are cleaned with cold water before hot water is used

    a. because hot water may coagulate the body secretions
    b. to kill certain microorganisms
    c. to economize on hot water
    d. to preserve the equipment

10. The nurse who is not familiar with equipment should

    a. try to figure out how it works
    b. not give the treatment at all
    c. ask for instructions and demonstration
    d. substitute another piece of equipment

11. Equipment should be handled with care because

    a. breakage would delay treatment needed by the patient
    b. defective equipment may injure the patient
    c. cost of repairs is expensive
    d. all of the above

12. Disposable equipment is desirable because

    a. it reduces the spread of infection
    b. its quality is superior
    c. it is cheaper than nondisposable equipment
    d. all of the above

B. Briefly answer the following questions.

1. Name the four environmental conditions which influence the patient's comfort.

2. State the difference between concurrent cleaning and terminal cleaning.

SECTION IV VITAL SIGNS AND ROUTINE CARE

unit 12 observing and recording

OBJECTIVES

After studying this unit, the student will be able to:

- Identify symptoms according to classification.
- Describe what information is contained in a chart.
- Define common charting abbreviations.

Careful observation and recording by the nurse are an important part of patient care. These techniques call the physician's attention to the patient's progress and responses to therapy. As the result of careful observations and reports, medications and treatments are often changed or discontinued. The nurse can add to the patient's well-being by making careful observations.

OBSERVING THE PATIENT

A symptom indicates disease or an abnormal condition. Some symptoms can be precisely measured while others cannot. Symptoms may be divided into three groups:

- *Subjective* symptoms are those which the patient experiences such as pain, weakness, and nausea.
- *Objective* symptoms are those which the nurse can observe such as swelling, inflammation, and vomiting.
- *Cardinal* symptoms are those which can be accurately measured such as temperature, pulse, respiration and blood pressure. These symptoms are sometimes called signs because they are measured objectively and are not personally experienced by the patient.

The nurse must be careful not to let her personal reactions interfere with her observation of the patient. It is important to listen to the patient. If the nurse is inattentive or hurried, the subjective symptoms may not be noticed. The patient may be uneasy about admitting to pain or weakness. The nurse must learn to allow patients to ask questions or express their needs. If patients can describe their own symptoms, the nurse can focus on the problem more quickly. Even though the questions seem irrelevant, the need for patients to ask them should be appreciated. The patient's anxiety may be the major cause of the illness, and the nurse can reduce it or even eliminate it by listening.

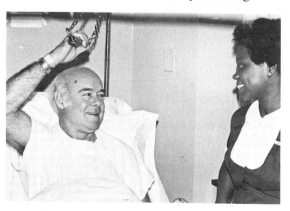

Fig. 12-1 Subjective symptoms may go unnoticed unless the nurse listens and observes carefully.

Since the nurse has the best opportunity to observe the patient, it is essential to be aware of what is considered normal and what might be an abnormal state. She must learn to watch carefully for changes and reactions in the patient and be able to recognize significant signs or symptoms. All symptoms which indicate a change in the patient's condition must be reported accurately and promptly.

Observation includes the use of all the senses. Changes in the color of the skin are seen. The nurse hears labored or irregular breathing. The sense of smell detects body odors which may be significant. Frequently, the patient describes his own symptoms and calls the nurse's attention to local pain or unusual sensitivity in a part of his body.

Many changes in the patient's condition can be detected and measured only by the use of one or more instruments. Those most frequently used are the thermometer for measuring temperature, the sphygmomanometer for determining blood pressure, chemicals for testing urine, graduated containers for measuring body intake and output, scales to weigh the patient and the rod to measure the patient's height.

Cardinal symptoms usually are measured with instruments or simple techniques. Measuring signs provides objective information. Little opinion or judgment is involved with the measurement. This factor is helpful in reducing error and confusion.

RECORDING PATIENT DATA

When a patient is admitted to the hospital, a chart is prepared. Chart forms vary with different health facilities. The chart provides a written record for the information relating to that patient. The chart includes the patient's personal data, admitting notes and history. As the patient receives care and

treatments, they are recorded. Laboratory studies, X-ray reports, and progress notes written by doctors and nurses are also included on the chart.

Writing notes in the patient's record is called *charting*. All charting must be accurate, brief, and clear. Facts — not opinions — are to be recorded. Only essential data should be entered on the chart and the notes should be clearly written. The use of accepted medical terms, symbols, and abbreviations will reduce confusion and avoid errors; notes should have the same meaning for all health team members.

Some abbreviations which are commonly used are:

a.c.	before meals
b.i.d.	twice a day
I. & O.	intake and output
I.V.	intravenous
p.o.	by mouth
p.r.n.	as needed
q.h.	every hour
stat	immediately

The chart must be readily identifiable. There should be absolutely no question about the relation of any chart to any patient. Page headings must have identifiable information about the patient. This always includes the name and room number, address, age, and other related information. Usually an addressograph is prepared when the patient is admitted and the plate imprint is made on each page as well as on the forms used for diagnostic tests (laboratory work, x-ray, etc.). The chart cover should be identified as well. Some covers already have room numbers marked on them but the patient's name should be inserted in the slot provided for it — as soon as possible. Patients should never be referred to by room number. Although many of the mechanics of chart preparation may be done by another person, the nurse is responsible for the care of the patient — this includes being sure the chart is accurately identified as well as being sure the charting is done properly.

VOCABULARY

- Define the following words:

abbreviations	continuous	subjective
cardinal	objective	symbols
classified	observation	symptom
confusion	precisely	terminology

SUGGESTED ACTIVITY

- Review the standard blank forms used for charting. Notice the difference between the progress notes for the doctors and the nurses. If possible, look at the addressograph and the information it prints on the paper.

REVIEW

A. Identify each of the following symptoms as subjective, objective or cardinal. Place the correct letter in front of each symptom.

S — subjective
O — objective
C — cardinal

_____ 1. pain
_____ 2. vomiting
_____ 3. nausea
_____ 4. body temperature
_____ 5. swelling

B. Briefly answer the following questions.

1. How do cardinal symptoms differ from other symptons?

2. Give four examples of the kind of information included in a patient's chart.

3. What should always be present on each page of the chart?

4. Name three rules or principles of good charting.

5. Define the following abbreviations:

a.c.

p.o.

p.r.n.

stat

unit 13 temperature

OBJECTIVES

After studying this unit, the student will be able to:

- Explain the importance of body temperature as an indicator of illness.
- Describe what is meant by body temperature.
- Compare an oral thermometer with a rectal thermometer, giving the advantages and disadvantages of each.
- Identify the steps to follow when taking and recording temperature.
- Recite the normal temperatures in Celsius (metric).

Temperature is the amount of heat in the body. It is the balance between heat production and heat loss. A change in body temperature is an important cardinal symptom. Often, a change in temperature is the first warning of a change in the patient's condition. A temperature change is an objective symptom measured by a thermometer. (Subjective and objective symptoms are differentiated in unit 12.)

Heat is lost by perspiring, exhaling, drinking cold liquids, and being exposed to cold. Heat is increased by exercise, external heat, and hot drinks. Infection causes an increase in temperature. Hemorrhage, starvation, or physical shock may cause a decrease in temperature. Variations in body temperature also occur normally throughout the day. In the evening the body is usually warmer than in the morning. Temperature varies in different areas of the body.

Large blood vessels that are located nearest the body surface are found in the mouth, axilla, groin and rectum. Placement of the thermometer near a large blood vessel is necessary if body temperature is to be measured. In the familiar glass thermometer, heat causes the mercury in the bulb to expand. The mercury then rises in the stem and a reading is obtained.

An electric thermometer saves time and reduces the spread of infection, figure 13-1, page 54. The thermometer registers in seconds, is accurate, and easy to read. When used orally, it provides an accurate reading even if the mouth is not closed. It is particularly useful for children and for adults who have breathing problems. Disposable covers fit over the end of the thermometer probe. This permits its optional use for oral or rectal readings, and eliminates the need for sterilization.

METHOD	USAGE	NORMAL TEMPERATURE
Oral	most convenient and most common	98.6°F (37°C)
Rectal	most accurate	99.2°F (37.3°C)
Axillary or groin	least accurate	97.6°F (36.4°C)

Glass thermometers must be sterilized. This takes time and is not always done carefully enough. In order to reduce the spread of infection, hospitals often issue one thermometer to be used by the patient. It is kept in the patient's unit during the entire hospital stay.

TAKING THE ORAL TEMPERATURE

Body temperature is taken orally when the patient can cooperate. An oral temperature is not taken when patients are unable to breathe through the nose; mouth breathing causes an inaccurate reading. An oral temperature is not taken if the patient has a history of convulsions. Infants and small children do not have temperatures taken with an oral thermometer. There is danger of physical injury because of restlessness and lack of attention. Moreover, the oral temperature is less accurate.

PROCEDURE

1. Assemble equipment near the bedside:

    Oral glass thermometer in a container
    Alcohol swabs or tissue

    Nurse should wear a watch with a second hand.

2. Greet patient and explain procedure.

    Do not take temperature if patient has taken hot or cold fluids within 10 minutes. Do not take temperature if patient is smoking or chewing gum.

3. Have patient rest in a comfortable position in the bed or chair.

    Washing the hands can be done while the patient is getting ready.

4. Remove thermometer from container by holding stem end. Read the mercury column. Check the condition of the thermometer.

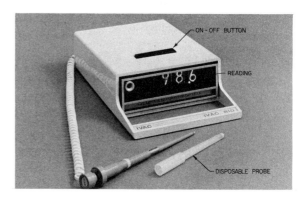

Fig. 13-1 An electronic thermometer gives a fast and accurate reading.

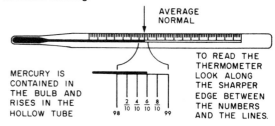

Fig. 13-2 The smallest mark on a Fahrenheit thermometer shows a tenth of a degree.

Never use a defective thermometer. If cracked or illegible, discard. If the thermometer has been standing in antiseptic solution, rinse it under cold water.

5. Wipe the thermometer with a tissue.

6. Shake the mercury down to at least 96°F (36°C).

7. Insert the bulb end of the thermometer under the patient's tongue, toward the side of the mouth. Ask the patient to hold the thermometer gently with lips closed.

    Do not touch the bulb of thermometer with the fingers. The patient should be reminded to breathe through the nose. He should not open his mouth until the thermometer has been removed.

8. Allow the thermometer to remain in place for 3 minutes.

    Stay with the patient if necessary.

9. Remove thermometer and wipe it with tissue.

   Hold the thermometer by the stem. Wipe from the stem end toward the bulb end.

10. Read the thermometer and record the temperature.

    Rotate the thermometer so that the mercury column can be seen clearly. Never guess at a reading. If reading does not appear accurate, retake temperature, using another thermometer.

11. Place the thermometer in its container and discard the wipe.

12. Record the temperature on the chart.
    Include: Time
             Procedure: *Temperature*
             Reading
             Observations

    Record as soon as possible. Report any unusual variation immediately to supervising nurse.

TAKING A RECTAL TEMPERATURE

A rectal thermometer differs slightly from the oral thermometer. On the rectal thermometer the end containing the mercury is short and more rounded, figure 13-3. The marks and numbers are the same on both thermometers. Rectal temperatures may be ordered by the doctor. When oral readings are not accurate, rectal readings must be taken. The nurse should not take a rectal temperature when a patient has diarrhea, a rectal problem, or rectal surgery. Patients placed under coronary precautions should not have rectal temperatures taken.

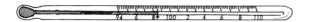

Fig. 13-3 The rectal thermometer has a rounded bulb for patient safety.

PROCEDURE

1. Assemble equipment as for oral temperature but include lubricant.

2. Greet patient and explain procedure; screen unit.

   Check the assignment to be sure the rectal temperature is ordered.

3. Lower the head of the bed, if the patient's condition permits. Ask the patient to turn on his side.

   Patient must be in the bed for this procedure. Assist if necessary.

4. Place a small amount of lubricant on a tissue.

5. Remove thermometer from container and shake the mercury down.

   Hold it by the stem end.

6. Apply a small amount of lubricant to the bulb.

   Use a downward movement toward the bulb.

7. Fold the top bedding back to expose the rectal area.

   Avoid exposing the patient to others. Use drapes if necessary.

8. Raise the upper buttock. Gently insert the thermometer into the rectum 3 cm (1 1/2 inches). Replace bedclothes as soon as thermometer is inserted.

   Insert thermometer gently with slight pressure; go past the sphincter muscle.

9. The thermometer should remain inserted for 3 to 5 minutes.

   Stay with the patient and hold the thermometer in place if necessary.

10. Remove the thermometer and wipe it thoroughly with a tissue or alcohol swab. Wipe toward the bulb.

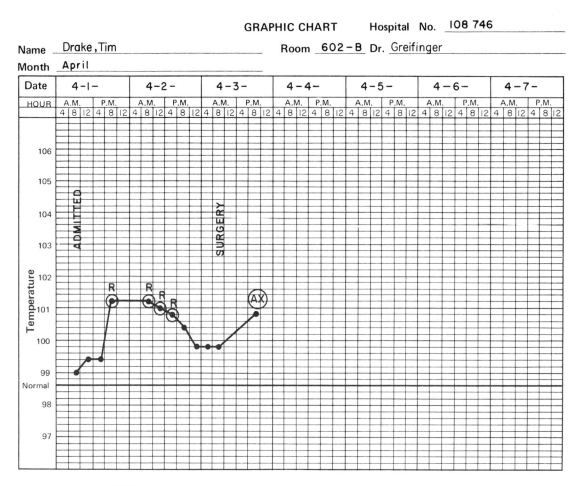

13-4 A properly-executed temperature chart should be informative.

Be sure to remove all organic matter. Clean again with a second swab if necessary.

11. Record the temperature and place an (R) next to the charted reading, figure 13-4.

VOCABULARY

- Define the following words:

antiseptic	coronary	probe
axillary	groin	shock
buttock	hemorrhage	sphincter
convulsions	lubricant	

SUGGESTED ACTIVITIES

- If a mannequin is available, practice taking a rectal temperature using the procedure described.
- Study and discuss the following topics:
    1. Objective symptoms of an elevated temperature.
    2. Nursing care usually advised for reducing fever.

- Obtain permission to visit a local hospital. Observe the variety of thermometers used. Which one is most commonly used?
- List conditions which may cause a decrease in temperature.

REVIEW

A. Briefly answer the following questions.

1. Why is the oral temperature taken more often that the rectal temperature?

2. When would it be dangerous to take a patient's temperature orally?

3. Name two advantages of the electronic thermometer.

4. How does a rectal thermometer differ from an oral thermometer?

5. Name four activities which would affect the reading of an oral thermometer.

6. Why is a change in body temperature an important sign?

7. When would you avoid taking a rectal temperature?

B.   Match the descriptions in column I with the correct terms in column II.

Column I

_____ 1. normal oral temperature in Celsius

_____ 2. normal rectal temperature in Celsius

_____ 3. activity which results in heat loss

_____ 4. activity which results in heat gain

_____ 5. time of day when body temperature is highest

_____ 6. a thermometer which registers temperature in seconds

_____ 7. length of time a rectal thermometer should be in place

_____ 8. the part of the thermometer to hold

_____ 9. length of time an oral thermometer should be in place

_____ 10. muscle around the rectum

Column II

a. exhaling
b. morning
c. 37°C
d. 98.6°C
e. 37.3°C
f. electronic
g. exercise
h. 3 to 5 minutes
i. evening
j. sphincter
k. bulb
l. 3 minutes
m. stem

unit 14 thermometer care

OBJECTIVES

After studying this unit, the student will be able to:

- Describe the steps used to clean and disinfect thermometers.
- Explain the advantages of having patients use and keep their own thermometers.

The thermometer is one of the most common measuring instruments used for patient care. Proper care of the thermometer is necessary so that it is clean and ready for use at any time.

Thermometers are contaminated after each use. Wiping with an alcohol swab may clean a thermometer but does not disinfect it. To be germfree, thermometers should be cleaned and disinfected. They must be cleaned with soap, water, and friction. To disinfect thermometers, most facilities require them to be soaked in a disinfectant solution. In most facilities, thermometer care becomes the duty of a nursing team member.

On admission, many facilities provide the patient with a thermometer and holder. The thermometer is used only by the patient throughout the hospital stay. This reduces the risk of spreading infections. Some facilities also allow patients to take the thermometer home with them. This policy saves the hospital time and money as the cleaning process is time-consuming and often results in breakage. In addition, there is the distinct advantage of eliminating the risk of cross-infection by using thermometers which might not have been properly disinfected.

PROCEDURE

1. Assemble equipment:
   Soap solution
   Disinfectant solution
   Thermometer holders
   Basin
   Cotton balls
   Soiled thermometers

2. Wash each thermometer separately with cotton balls and soap solution. Clean from stem to bulb end. Rinse in cold running water.

   Rotate the thermometer while cleaning it to be sure all organic matter is removed. Also, friction is a mechanical way of destroying some kinds of bacteria.

3. Place the thermometer in disinfectant solution.

   Make sure thermometers are completely covered with solution.

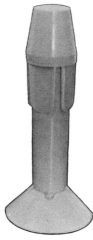

Fig. 14-1 A bedside holder keeps the thermometer clean and protected.

4. Place a label on the basin to show what time the thermometers may be used.

Thirty minutes in disinfectant is the time specified by many hospitals.

5. Clean each thermometer holder and place cotton in the bottom.

6. After the specified time has passed, remove the thermometers from the disinfectant solution. Rinse with cold water. Examine for breakage.

7. Shake mercury down in each thermometer.

If a shaker is used, hold thermometers carefully and securely.

8. Place thermometers in the clean holders.

Handle carefully to avoid breakage.

9. Replace cleaning equipment. Discard used cotton balls and solutions.

VOCABULARY

- Define the following words:

  disinfectant   eliminate   cross-infection

SUGGESTED ACTIVITIES

- Practice the procedure described for cleaning a thermometer. Follow the steps as outlined until you can demonstrate thermometer care for your instructor's evaluation.

- Discuss reasons why cold water is used to clean thermometers before they are disinfected.

REVIEW

Briefly answer the following questions.

1. In what direction should the contaminated thermometer be wiped?

2. In the course of one day, how often does the thermometer become contaminated?

3. In most facilities, who is responsible for thermometer care?

4. Why should thermometers be rotated during cleaning?

5. What advantage is it to allow patients to keep their thermometers?

unit 15 pulse

OBJECTIVES

After studying this unit, the student will be able to:

- Define pulse.
- Identify body sites where the pulse can be taken.
- Name three factors that are to be noted when taking the pulse.
- List the possible causes for changes in pulse rate.
- Describe how to take the radial pulse.

Pulse is the alternate expansion and contraction of an artery caused by the contractions of the heart forcing blood through the artery. The pulse reflects the heartbeat and is an important indicator of how the heart is working. Pulse is present in every artery of the body but is best detected where the artery is close to a bone, figure 15-1.

The pulse is usually taken over the radial artery on the wrist where it can be easily felt. In some patients it may be necessary to take an apical pulse. A stethoscope is placed over the tip (apex) of the patient's heart, just below the left nipple. The stethoscope enables the nurse to hear the pulse. The pulse is taken by counting the heartbeats, at the apex, while listening with the stethoscope.

The doctor may ask the nurse to take both the radial and apical pulse. The pulse rate may be different in the two areas when the patient has blood flow problems. The difference between the radial pulse and the apical pulse is called the *pulse deficit*. Arteriosclerosis (loss of elasticity of the blood vessels) often causes a pulse deficit.

The pulse rate varies with a number of factors. Age, sex, and size of the patient are natural factors which influence the pulse rate. Increase in the pulse rate occurs with exercise, eating, emotional responses, and extremes of heat and cold. Drugs which are stimulants and foods, such as coffee and tea, may also increase pulse rate. Decrease in the pulse rate occurs with fasting, rest or sleep, and drugs which act as depressants. Quiet, stable emotions and mild temperatures keep the pulse rate steady.

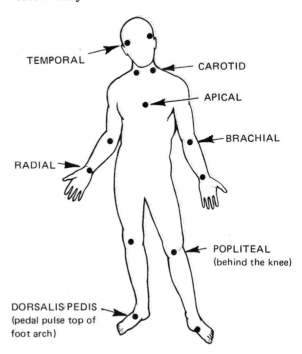

TEMPORAL
CAROTID
APICAL
BRACHIAL
RADIAL
POPLITEAL
(behind the knee)
DORSALIS PEDIS
(pedal pulse top of
foot arch)

Fig. 15-1 Many areas of the body can be used to obtain the pulse.

┌─────────────── AVERAGE PULSE RATES ───────────────┐

60– 90 beats per minute for adults

70– 90 beats per minute for children over 7 years

80–120 beats per minute for children 1–7 years

110–130 beats per minute for infants

125–155 beats per minute for the fetus

└───┘

When taking the pulse, the nurse should note:

- Rate: number of beats per minute
- Rythym: regular, irregular
- Volume: strong, weak

A rapid heart rate is called *tachycardia*. A slow heart rate is called *bradycardia*. An irregular rate is called an arrhythmia. All are extremes and show an abnormal condition. They should always be reported to the charge nurse.

PROCEDURE FOR TAKING THE RADIAL PULSE

1. Greet the patient.

2. Place patient in a comfortable position. The palm of his hand should be down and his arm supported.

   The patient should be sitting down or lying in bed when the pulse is being taken. The patient's arm may rest on his chest.

3. Locate the pulse on the thumb side of the patient's wrist. Use the tips of the first three fingers, not the thumb, figure 15-2.

   By using the thumb, the nurse's own pulse would be felt instead of the patient's pulse.

4. When the pulse is felt, exert slight pressure and count for 1 minute.

   Use the second hand of the watch. The pulse can be counted for 30 seconds and multiplied by 2 to obtain a one minute rate. However, counting for one full minute is preferred.

5. Record the rate, rhythm and volume of the pulse on the patient's chart. Pulse rate can also be marked on a graph with the temperature, figure 15-3.

   Report any unusual observations to the charge nurse.

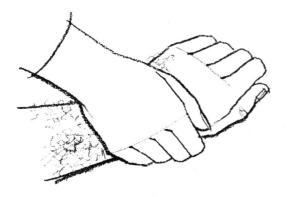
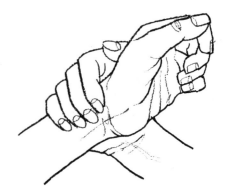

Fig. 15-2 Always use the tips of the fingers to feel the radial pulse.

U.S. GOVERNMENT PRINTING OFFICE: 1961 0—602627

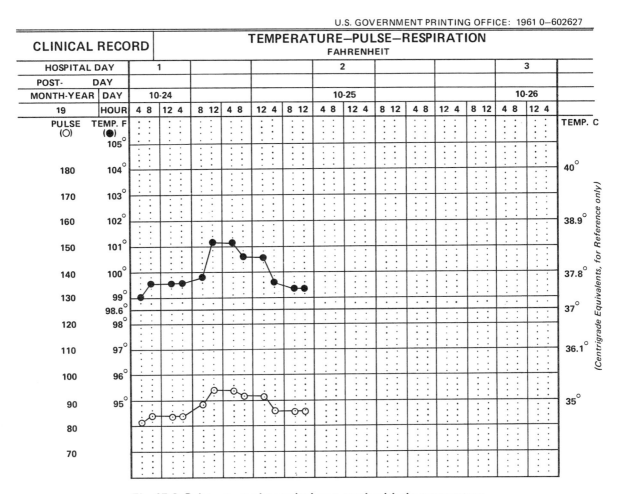

Fig. 15-3 Pulse rate can be marked on a graph with the temperature.

VOCABULARY

- Define the following words:

apical	depressant	radial
arrhythmic	dorsal pedis	rhythm
arteriosclerosis	expansion	stethoscope
brachial	facial	stimulant
bradycardia	femoral	tachycardia
carotid	popliteal	temporal
contraction	pulse deficit	

SUGGESTED ACTIVITIES

- Practice taking the radial pulse of another student. Compare the rates of two or three other students.

- Observe the effect that exercise has on the pulse rate. Ask another student to run in place for one minute. Compare the pulse before and after.

REVIEW

Briefly answer the following questions.

1. Name three natural factors that determine a person's general pulse rate.

2. List four factors that increase pulse rate.

3. What is the average pulse rates for the following?
   a. Adult: _____ to _____ beats per minute
   b. Child (1-7 years): _____ to _____ beats per minute

4. Define the following terms:
   a. tachycardia

   b. bradycardia

   c. pulse

   d. arrhythmia

5. What three factors should the nurse note about the pulse?

6. Where is the apical pulse taken? Give the exact location.

7. When taking a radial pulse, why must the nurse avoid resting her thumb on the patient's wrist?

8. What is the pulse deficit?

9. Where can the brachial pulse be found?

10. Describe the way to take a radial pulse.

unit 16 respiration

OBJECTIVES

After studying this unit, the student will be able to:

- State the main function of respiration.
- Explain how to count respirations.
- State the normal respiration rate for adults.
- Recognize and define terms which describe breathing problems.

The main function of respiration is to supply the cells in the body with oxygen and to remove carbon dioxide. Respiration is a sign of life. Therefore, it is observed along with the other vital signs.

Respirations must be counted while the patient is not aware of it. Otherwise the patient may breathe differently and alter the normal rate. One respiration includes the complete rise and fall of the chest. The rate includes all respirations for one minute. The nurse should count using a watch with a second hand. The normal respiration rate for adults is 14 to 18 per minute. If the rate is over 25 per minute it is said to be *accelerated*.

Respiration quality should also be noted. The rhythm may be irregular or have a *Cheyne-Stokes* rate. This is deep breathing which is interrupted by periods of shallow breathing or no breathing at all. The absence of respiration is called *apnea*. Difficult or labored breathing is called *dyspnea*. Pain usually occurs with dyspnea. If a patient must sit or stand erect in order to breath, the condition is called *orthopnea*. In these cases, it is necessary to raise the head of the bed or place the patient in a sitting position. The overbed table can be utilized by the patient who must sleep in the sitting position.

Cyanosis may occur with abnormal respiratory conditions. *Cyanosis* is the bluish color of the skin which results when the bloodstream does not receive enough oxygen. Cyanosis first appears in the lips and in the nail beds as a sign of oxygen lack. If the low level of oxygen persists, dizziness and loss of consciousness results.

PROCEDURE

1. Have the patient sit or lie down. Position your hands to appear as if the pulse were to be taken.

   If the pulse has just been counted, leave the fingers on the wrist. In this way the patient is not aware that his breathing rate is being taken.

2. Count the number of times the chest rises and falls during one minute.

   If necessary, some of the bedding may be folded down, so the chest movements can be easily seen. Be sure the patient is not exposed.

3. If chest movements are too slight to see, lay the patient's arm over the chest and begin counting again, figure 16-1, page 66.

   This can be done while feeling the radial pulse.

4. Observe the respirations for depth and regularity.

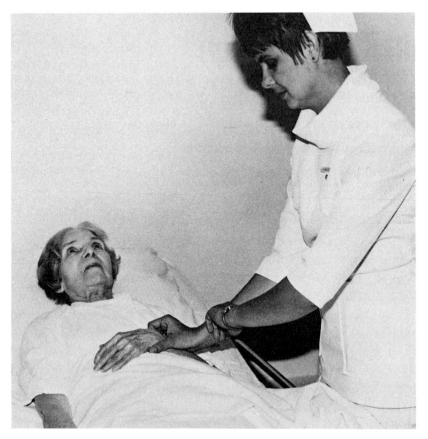

Fig. 16-1 Placing the patient's arm over her chest helps the nurse count the breathing movements.

Look for facial expressions which may indicate that breathing is painful.

5. Record the respiration rate on the same sheet with the temperature and pulse. Record the quality if it is abnormal.

Note any difficulty or cyanosis observed. Report unusual observations to the charge nurse immediately.

VOCABULARY

- Define the following words:

accelerated	consciousness	oxygen
apnea	cyanosis	respiration
carbon dioxide	dyspnea	vital
Cheyne-Stokes	orthopnea	

SUGGESTED ACTIVITIES

- Practice counting respirations with other students: have two students count respirations of a third student at the same time. Compare rates of respiration. Retake respirations after student has run in place. Note and discuss the change.

- Using outside sources, write a brief paragraph on each of the following topics:

    1. How respiration is regulated and controlled

    2. Three types of illness which increase respirations

    3. Common symptoms of respiratory difficulty

REVIEW

Briefly answer the following questions.

1. What is the normal respiration rate for an adult?

2. Why should the patient be unaware of the fact that the respirations are being counted?

3. What is the main function of respiration?

4. What movements are included in one complete respiration?

5. What happens to the skin when there is a decrease in the oxygen level?

6. Describe a Cheyne-Stokes respiration.

7. What is the difference between dyspnea and orthopnea?

8. Name two ways to better observe chest movements when counting a patient's respirations.

9. Where does cyanosis first appear as a sign that the oxygen level is low?

10. How long does the nurse count to obtain the respiration rate?

unit 17 blood pressure

OBJECTIVES

After studying this unit, the student will be able to:

- Define blood pressure.
- Differentiate between systolic and diastolic pressure.
- List physical conditions which affect blood pressure.
- Describe the procedure for taking the blood pressure.
- State the meaning of pulse pressure.

Blood pressure is one of the vital signs. It is the force of blood against the walls of the blood vessels. When the heart beats, blood is forced out of the heart. This is the phase when the pressure in the blood vessels is the highest. The reading taken at this point is the *systolic* blood pressure. When the heart rests between beats, blood returns to the heart from the veins. This is the *diastolic* blood pressure. It is the time when least force is exerted against the walls of the blood vessels.

Blood pressure is measured with a sphygmomanometer and a stethoscope. This equipment is needed since blood pressure cannot be heard without it. The *sphygmomanometer* has (1) a cuff for the patient's arm, (2) a rubber air bulb, (3) a control valve to release the air, and (4) a gauge which gives the reading.

Blood pressure is affected by a number of factors. Two of these factors are the volume of blood in circulation, and the strength of the heartbeat. The condition of the arteries also greatly affects the blood pressure. Arteries which have lost their elasticity or have become narrow because of deposits, make it more difficult for the blood to flow. Greater force is needed to push the blood through the arteries; this increases the blood pressure.

Temporary changes in blood pressure vary with daily activities. Increases occur with exercise, eating, becoming excited or upset, and taking stimulants. Decreases occur with fasting, physical or mental rest, and the use of depressants.

PROCEDURE

1. Assemble equipment:

   Sphygmomanometer
   Stethoscope

2. Greet the patient and explain the procedure.

3. Support the left arm with palm of the hand facing upward on the bed or table.

   The left brachial artery is usually used so that readings will be uniform. There is a slight difference between the readings of the right and left arm.

4. Roll the sleeve of the gown up about 5 inches above the elbow.

5. Apply the cuff above the elbow and directly over the brachial artery.

   The two tubes from the cuff should rest over the inside bend of the elbow.

6. Wrap the rest of the armband smoothly around the arm.

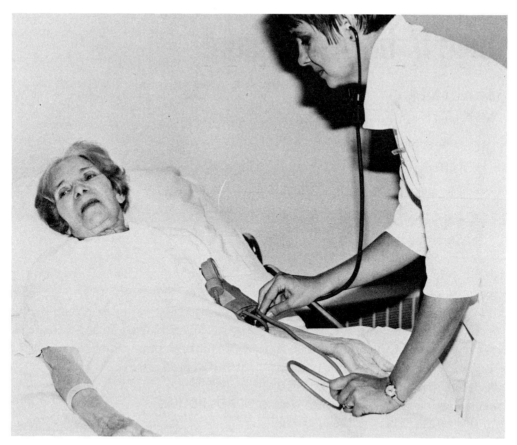

Fig. 17-1 The patient must lie still in order for the nurse to hear the pulse sounds.

7. Locate the brachial artery with the fingers. Place the stethoscope directly over the artery. Place earpieces in ears.

   No sound will be heard but the pulse can be felt.

8. Close the valve attached to the air bulb and inflate the cuff. Stop when the gauge registers at least *150,* or 20 millimeters above the point where the pulse is no longer heard.

   As the cuff tightens, it presses on the artery, closing it. The pulse sounds cease abruptly when the artery is completely closed.

9. Slowly open the valve and let air escape until the first sound is heard.

10. At this first sound, note the reading on the gauge. This is the systolic pressure.

11. Continue to release the air until there is an abrupt change in sound from loud to soft. The reading at which this change is heard is the diastolic pressure.

    Noise or movement may interfere with the reading and require that the blood pressure be retaken. If this occurs, deflate the cuff, wait 15 seconds and begin again.

12. Blood pressure readings which seem abnormal or are difficult to hear should be rechecked.

    Have another team member retake the blood pressure if necessary.

13. Remove cuff, expel the air, and replace the equipment.

14. Record the blood pressure as a fraction. For example 120/80 means that

120 is the systolic pressure and 80 is the diastolic pressure. The *pulse pressure* is the difference between the systolic and diastolic pressures. In this case it is 40.

Report abnormal readings immediately to the charge nurse. Be alert to readings which are different from those normally shown for the patient.

VOCABULARY

- Define the following words:

deposits	inflate	systolic
diastolic	pulse pressure	valve
gauge	sphygmomanometer	volume

SUGGESTED ACTIVITIES

- Practice taking blood pressure readings with another student. Compare the readings taken while the other student is: 1. lying down 2. sitting in a chair 3. resting after much activity.

REVIEW

Briefly answer the following questions.

1. What is blood pressure?

2. Describe the heart action which produces the systolic and diastolic blood pressure.

3. Name the four major parts of a sphygmomanometer.

4. List four common causes of a temporary increase in blood pressure.

5. List three factors that may permanently affect the blood pressure.

6. Over which artery is the stethoscope placed when taking blood pressure?

7. When placing the cuff on the arm, where should the two tubes rest?

8. What pressure is represented by the first sound heard after the cuff has been inflated and the valve opened.

9. How long must the nurse wait to retake the blood pressure if she is unsure of the reading?

10. What is pulse pressure?

unit 18 intake and output

OBJECTIVES

After studying this unit, the student will be able to:

- Define fluid balance.

- Name the two major areas where body fluids may be found.

- List four causes of dehydration.

- List different kinds of output.

- Identify steps used to measure and record intake and output.

Two-thirds of the body weight is water. Knowing the amount of fluid taken in and eliminated is important. Certain disorders require the doctor to know the patient's exact intake and output. Nurses have an important role in keeping this record.

FLUID BALANCE

When the body's intake of fluid equals its output, the body is in *fluid balance*. Normally, the amount of fluid taken into the body during a 24-hour period is about 2600 milliliters. Fluid not absorbed by the body is excreted as urine and perspiration. The body maintains a fluid balance using processes which are quite complex. Body fluid is found in two major areas: inside the cells (intracellular) and outside the cells (extracellular). The chemical balance is chiefly maintained by the urinary system.

In illness, the difference between fluid intake and output may be large. One type of fluid imbalance occurs when excess fluid is retained in the body. This is called *edema*; it may be general or local. *Ascites,* a collection of fluid in the peritoneal cavity, is an example of edema.

Excessive loss of fluid may be the result of vomiting, diarrhea, hemorrhage or *diaphoresis* (profuse sweating). Dehydration re-

sults when the loss is too great and the intake is not enough to make up for the loss. This can lead to a serious state of fluid imbalance. The kidneys cannot remove toxins from the bloodstream without proper amounts of fluid. Lowered body temperature, weakness, and eventually stupor follow prolonged loss of fluid.

RECORDING INTAKE AND OUTPUT

An accurate recording of intake and output is part of the care of many hospital patients. The doctor may want a record of the patient's daily intake and output to help diagnose or plan treatment. Intake and output, (I. & O.) is required for patients who are receiving intravenous fluids and who have indwelling urinary catheters. Catheters are used to guide urine flow from the bladder into a collection bag where it can be measured, figure 18-1, page 74. The catheter provides relief to the patient who has a urinary problem. When a catheter and bag are not used, a graduated pitcher is used to measure urine.

The metric system is most often used for measuring fluids. The nurse should become familiar with metric units. A milliliter is similar to a cubic centimeter. However, milliliter is more appropriate to use as it refers to capacity (fluid or liquid) while cubic centimeter refers to volume (air or gas).[1] Most hospital equipment is still marked in cubic centimeters.

PROCEDURE

Recording Intake

1. Gather supplies:

   Intake and output record
   Graduated pitcher

2. Review the I. & O. record with the patient. Discuss the amount and kind of fluids taken.

   Patients should take part in keeping their own records. Sometimes visitors or the patient may forget to record fluids drunk by him.

3. Use the graduated pitcher to measure fluids left in cups or glasses. Subtract the amount left from the amount the container usually holds.

Example

Coffee cup capacity	120 ml
Amount of coffee left	20 ml
Intake	100 ml

4. Record: Fluids taken with meals
   Amount of fluids taken between meals
   Fluids given with medications
   I.V. fluids
   Tube feedings

5. Use the correct method of recording according to hospital policy. Be sure to include the date, time, method of administration, type and amount of fluid. Some hospitals require I. & O. to be recorded both at the bedside and on the patient's chart, figure 18-3.

6. Total the intake for the 24-hour period as established by hospital policy. Usually the time is 12 A.M. (midnight) or 6 A.M. The total is always recorded on the patient's chart.

Example

I.V.	3000 ml
p.o.	2000 ml
	5000 ml TOTAL

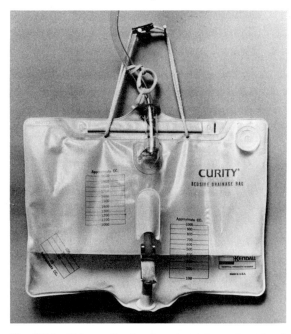

Fig. 18-1 Urine collection bags hang from the side of the bed and collect urine which flows through the tubing.

Household measures		Milliliters (cubic centimeters)
1 teaspoon	=	4
1 fluid ounce	=	30
1 juice glass	=	100
1 coffee cup	=	120
1 eight ounce glass	=	240
1 pint	=	500
1 quart	=	1000

Fig. 18-2 Learning the approximate equivalents helps the nurse in recording I. & O.

1. *Tabor's Cyclopedic Medical Dictionary*, 13th ed., App. 7

FLUID INTAKE AND OUTPUT

Name _Smith, Frederick W._   Room _525 B_

Date	Time	Method of Adm.	INTAKE		OUTPUT				
			Solution	mL Amounts Received	Time	mL Urine Amount	OTHERS		
							Kind	Amount	
4/13	7 A.M.	p.o.	milk, coffee juice	540	6 A.M.	500	liquid stool	100	
	10:15	I.V.	D/W	840	11:00	400			
	12:00	p.o.	soup riced tea	480	4 P.M.	700	vomitus	20	
	3 P.M.	p.o.	water	60					
	5:00	p.o.	milk, juice	645	7:00	300			
	9:00	p.o.	coke + water	120	10:30	600			

Methods of Administration

p.o.   oral or by mouth
I.V.   intraveneous
TF   tube feeding

Fig. 18-3 Intake and Output records are usually kept at the bedside.

Recording Output

1. Gather supplies:

   Intake and output record
   Graduated pitcher
   Bedpan or urinal

2. Ask patient to use bedpan or urinal, and avoid dropping toilet paper into the urine. Pour the urine into the graduated pitcher to measure it.

3. Ambulatory patients must use a bedpan or urinal when their output is to be recorded.

   Nurses may have to remind these patients _not_ to use the toilet. Some patients can be taught to measure their own urine. Be sure the patient is able and willing to measure carefully.

4. Check whether the patient has a catheter and collection bag. If so, empty the bag and measure the urine in the graduated pitcher.

5. Observe the urine for presence of blood, pus, or particles. Note the color and odor. Report any changes which seem abnormal.

6. Record the amount measured and any unusual observations.

   If part of the urine is lost, estimate the amount and note that the loss occurred.

7. Record other liquid output.

   Vomitus, liquid stool, wound drainage, fluid aspirated from the stomach

or other body cavities, and perspiration must all be considered. Perspiration and wound drainage may be described as little, moderate, or excessive.

8. Rinse the graduated pitcher with cold water. Clean and replace it according to hospital policy.

9. Transfer information from intake and output record to the patient's chart according to hospital policy.

VOCABULARY

- Define the following words:

ambulatory	diaphoresis	intake
ascites	edema	output
aspirated	equivalent	profuse
catheter	excreted	stupor
cavities	fluid balance	toxin
dehydration	graduate	urinary system

SUGGESTED ACTIVITY

- Using outside sources as reference, study the methods commonly used to increase a patient's fluid intake. Discuss your findings with the class.

REVIEW

Briefly answer the following questions.

1. What fraction of total body weight consists of water?

2. Name the two major areas where body fluid is found.

3. Name the body system that is chiefly responsible for maintaining fluid balance.

4. Name four causes of dehydration.

5. How does an inadequate fluid level affect kidney function?

6. Define fluid balance.

7. For how many hours is intake and output recorded before the sum is totaled?

8. Name three sources of fluids which should be included as intake.

9. Name five kinds of fluid output.

10. What is used for measuring fluid output?

unit 19 admitting and discharging the patient

OBJECTIVES

After studying this unit, the student will be able to:

- Identify principles for admitting or discharging a patient.
- Explain the procedure for admitting a patient.
- Explain the procedure for discharging a patient.
- List observations which should be reported.

The nurse is responsible for the patient's safety and care during an admission, transfer, or discharge. Other health team members or hospital staff personnel help with these procedures. However, the nurse must see that details are carried through correctly and that the comfort of the patient is of primary concern.

Even before the patient is admitted to a hospital, the necessity for the hospitalization usually worries the patient. The family and friends may also be concerned and may demand much of the attention. The nurse must be especially aware of the anxiety and try to relieve it by creating a favorable impression. Being kind and confident gains the trust and cooperation of others. If the visitors must be asked to leave, the nurse should do so kindly in a firm but polite manner.

ADMISSION

Usually the clerk in the admitting office will call the floor nurse after the admission interview has been completed and the patient is ready to be brought to his or her room. If information about the manner of admission — ambulatory or by ambulance — has not been provided, the nurse should ask about it and whether any special equipment will be needed. A volunteer or aide often accompanies the patient and carries personal data which will become part of the chart. If the patient is brought from the emergency room, the data may be more complete as the patient will have been seen by a physician and orders written. Usually, the floor nurse is notified beforehand if the patient is going to need oxygen therapy, siderails, and any special equipment. This is done so that arrangements can be made to make the transfer safely and smoothly for the patient with as little discomfort as possible.

ADMISSION PROCEDURE

1. Assemble supplies and equipment.

   Urine specimen container
   Thermometer and holder
   Stethoscope
   Admission information form
   Sphygmomanometer

2. Prepare the unit by making sure that all necessary equipment and furniture are in the proper places. Check for adequate lighting and ventilation. Open the bed by fanfolding the covers.

3. Greet the patient. The nurse should introduce herself and check the patient's identification.

   Refer to the ID Bracelet and repeat the name. Do not appear to rush the patient. Be kind and helpful to the patient and his family.

4. Ask the family to wait in the lounge or lobby while the patient is getting ready for bed. Introduce the patient to the others in the room. Explain the call signal system. Insofar as it is permitted, explain the routine procedures that are likely to happen in the next hour.

If the patient seems to be tired or weak, help him into bed immediately.

5. Screen the unit for privacy.

6. Help the patient to undress and to put on a gown. Care for personal clothing according to hospital policy.

Respect the patient's modesty and need for privacy.

7. If the patient is able to walk about, take the height and weight.

Even if the patient knows his weight, weigh him anyway. Illness often causes a weight change the patient may not notice.

8. Help the patient get into bed. Adjust the siderails if ordered.

9. Make a list of any belongings, jewelry or valuables that the patient wants to keep in the room. Ask the patient to sign the list. This protects the hospital and health team members. Relatives should also sign the list, and valuables should be taken home if possible. Money or valuables that must stay should be kept in the hospital safe.

10. Tell the patient that a urine specimen is needed and offer the bedpan or urinal.

Assist the patient as necessary. Do not leave a weak patient alone.

11. Prepare the urine specimen as instructed. Clean and replace the bedpan or urinal.

Be sure to label the specimen correctly.

12. Take the patient's temperature, pulse, respiration and blood pressure. Clean and replace equipment used.

Report abnormal vital signs to the charge nurse. Thermometers and sphygmomanometers should always be ready for future use.

13. Observe the patient's condition while caring for him. Note the condition of his skin. Check for rashes, cuts, scratches, discoloration, or the presence of lice. Observe for loss of motion in the limbs and signs of weakness or pain. Note whether the patient is mentally alert.

Be tactful and discreet in observation. Report immediately any observations which you judge to be significant.

14. Encourage the patient to lie down and rest. Place the signal cord within reach. Provide fresh drinking water. Remove screen. Tell relatives they may visit the patient.

On admission, the patient may have to stay in or near the room to wait for the doctor's first visit.

15. Record the admission on the Nursing Notes, figure 19-1, page 80. Be sure the chart contains the following information.

    Name of patient
    Room number and bed
    Doctor's name
    Date and time of admission
    Method of admission
    Age, height, weight, sex
    T.P.R. and B/P
    Patient's complaints about illness
    Signs and symptoms observed

NAME _____ Gonzalez, Gilbert _____

ROOM _____ 211A _____

DOCTOR _____ Reyna _____

	CLINICAL RECORD		NURSING NOTES
Date	HOUR		OBSERVATIONS
	A.M.	P.M.	
9-1-79		4:00 P.M.	Male, 65 yr. old admitted in a wheelchair. Height 5'8" and weight 165 lbs. Vital Signs - temp. 37.2°C orally pulse 84 resp. 20 B/P 130/90 Urine specimen collected 150ml and sent to lab. Abdomen distended and patient complaining of cramping – Dr. Reyna notified. a. Wool, LPN

Fig. 19-1 Admission notes should be complete and clear.

Collection and description of specimen

Signature of health team member writing report

In most agencies, the chart may be assembled by the ward clerk. An addressograph may be used to complete parts of the chart (name, hospital number, etc.).

DISCHARGE

The discharge of any patient needs the written order of the physician. A discharge should be organized and well planned. Often the patient may need to know about new medicines, dressings, or a diet change. The patient must be taught self-care before the day of discharge.

Discharge plans may include use of other services outside the hospital. These plans are called referrals. The patient may be referred to a public health nurse, social worker, or doctor who is a specialist. Referrals require a doctor's order.

Discharge from the hospital may be a joy or a hardship for the patient. The recovering patient may find it hard to adjust to another setting. The nurse should be aware that each patient has a different home life. Some patients will need more help with discharge planning than others. In order to save time and prevent stress for the patient on the day of discharge, a relative may go to the business office and take care of the financial arrangements. Needless stress for the patient should be avoided.

DISCHARGE PROCEDURE

1. Check to be sure the patient's discharge has been ordered by the doctor.

If the patient and/or his name is unfamiliar, check the identification (ID) bracelet to avoid error.

2. Take a wheelchair to the patient's room.

   Most hospitals require the use of a wheelchair, even when the patient is able to walk.

3. Greet the patient and discuss the discharge plans.

   Be alert to the patient's feelings about leaving.

4. Screen the unit and help the patient to dress if necessary.

5. Collect the personal belongings and help with any necessary packing.

   Check valuables against the list made on admission. Make sure that all of the patient's belongings have been removed from the closet and bedside stand.

6. Tell the patient (or a member of his family) how to collect valuables from the hospital safe and where to go to make the necessary financial arrangements.

7. Help patient into the wheelchair.

8. Escort the patient to the discharge area of the hospital. Help the patient into the car.

   Never accept tips for these or any other services.

9. Return wheelchair. Strip hospital unit. Clean and replace equipment used in care of patient. Ventilate the unit.

10. Record: Date and time of discharge
    Use of wheelchair or stretcher
    Observations as to the apparent condition of patient

VOCABULARY

- Define the following words:

admission	discoloration	referral
ambulatory	discreet	stress
ambulance	escort	tactful
discharge	lice	valuables

SUGGESTED ACTIVITIES

- Investigate the admission procedure of a local hospital.
- Role play admitting a patient to the hospital unit. Record the necessary information on the patient's chart. Have another student evaluate your technique.
- Discuss hospital procedures for patients who decide to leave against the advice of the physician.

REVIEW

A. Select the *best* answer.

1. The admitting nurse may help put the patient at ease by
   a. leaving the patient and letting him find his way around
   b. introducing him to other patients in the room and explaining the call light signal
   c. asking relatives and friends to leave and telling them the visiting hours
   d. speaking softly

2. The best place for the patient's own clothing is

    a. in the closet   c. in the hospital safe
    b. in the drawers   d. home with the family

3. Procedures carried out by the nurse upon admission of a patient include

    a. measuring the height and weight
    b. taking the vital signs
    c. collecting a urine specimen
    d. all of the above

4. On admission the nurse observes the patient for

    a. weakness   c. lice
    b. signs of pain   d. all of the above

5. Cleaning the unit following a discharge involves

    a. ventilating the room and stripping the bed
    b. making an open bed and leaving the room for the housekeeping department to clean
    c. replacing used equipment and making an open bed
    d. closing the door and notifying the charge nurse the room is empty

6. When discharging the patient, the nurse should

    a. escort the patient to the elevator
    b. go to the business office to settle the patient's bill
    c. teach the patient about self-care
    d. check to see that the doctor ordered the discharge

7. The nurse can gain the cooperation of visitors by using a manner which is

    a. brisk and efficient   c. firm but polite
    b. hurried   d. meek

8. Teaching a patient about new self-care should be done

    a. at a time when the doctor is present
    b. when the nursing education department can assist
    c. before the day the patient is to be discharged
    d. only after the patient is resting at home

B. Briefly answer the following questions.

1. Name four things that should be recorded at the time a patient is admitted.

2. Name three things that should be recorded at the time the patient is discharged.

SELF-EVALUATION IV

A. Select the *best* answer.

1. When a patient is admitted, the nurse should record
   a. the method of admission
   b. observations of the nurse
   c. vital signs
   d. all of the above

2. Before a patient is discharged, it is essential that
   a. the patient is ambulatory
   b. a doctor's discharge order is written
   c. medications are given for the patient to take home
   d. a nurse is available for home care

3. A rectal temperature should not be taken when the patient
   a. is obese
   b. is in a coma
   c. has diarrhea
   d. is elderly

4. The length of time an oral temperature must be left in place is
   a. four minutes
   b. five minutes
   c. three minutes
   d. one minute

5. The length of time the rectal thermometer must be left in place is about
   a. five minutes
   b. two minutes
   c. one minute
   d. six minutes

6. Body temperature is increased by
   a. perspiration
   b. infection
   c. exposure to cold
   d. expiration of air

7. The artery most frequently used in taking the patient's pulse is the
   a. facial
   b. temporal
   c. carotid
   d. radial

8. The pulse rate is increased by
   a. exercise
   b. fasting
   c. depressants
   d. rest

9. The part of a sphygmomanometer which controls the release of air is the
   a. cuff
   b. stethoscope
   c. gauge
   d. valve

10. An intake record may include
    a. tube feedings, vomitus, and snacks
    b. urine, liquid stool, and perspiration
    c. tube feedings, I.V. fluids, and water between meals
    d. I.V. fluids, tube feedings and catheterized urine

11. Intake and output is recorded when

    a. an indwelling catheter is in place
    b. the patient is receiving intravenous fluids
    c. the doctor orders it
    d. all of the above

12. One fluid ounce is equal to

    a. 30 milliliters   c. 200 milliliters
    b. 1 liter   d. 100 milliliters

13. An excessive loss of body fluid may result in

    a. edema   c. ascites
    b. stupor   d. sweating

14. Normal breathing is called

    a. dyspnea   c. Cheyne-Stokes
    b. respiration   d. orthopnea

15. The vital signs are

    a. blood pressure and pulse
    b. temperature, pulse, and respirations
    c. temperature, pulse, respirations, and blood pressure
    d. respirations and blood pressure

B. Briefly answer the following questions.

 1. Define three classifications of symptoms and give one example of each.

 2. Name kinds of information included in a patient's chart.

 3. Give the medical abbreviations for the following terms:

    a. twice a day

    b. intravenous

    c. by mouth

    d. every hour

 4. State the normal oral temperature in Celsius and Fahrenheit.

5. Give the range for the average pulse rate of an adult.

6. What is the normal rate of respiration per minute for adults?

7. Name two advantages in using the electronic thermometer.

8. What two separate pieces of equipment are used to take blood pressure?

9. What current system of measurement should be used for measuring and totalling fluids?

10. Which health team member gives permission for the discharge of a patient?

C. Match the definitions in Column I with the correct terms in Column II.

Column I

Column II

_____ 1. rapid heart rate

_____ 2. excess fluid in the peritoneal cavity

_____ 3. the difference between the systolic and the diastolic pressure

_____ 4. the difference between the radial pulse and the apical pulse

_____ 5. bluish skin tone caused by insufficient oxygen

_____ 6. profuse sweating

_____ 7. abnormally slow heart rate

_____ 8. blood pressure reading while the heart is at rest

_____ 9. the absence of respiration

_____ 10. medical abbreviation for immediately

_____ 11. when the body's fluid intake and output are equal

_____ 12. blood pressure reading when pressure in the blood vessels is at its highest

_____ 13. excess fluid retained in the body

_____ 14. pulse with irregular rhythm

_____ 15. difficult breathing

a. apnea

b. bradycardia

c. pulse deficit

d. diaphoresis

e. systolic

f. arrhythmic

g. ascites

h. tachycardia

i. stat

j. edema

k. dyspnea

l. fluid balance

m. pulse pressure

n. diastolic

o. cyanosis

SECTION V ASSISTING WITH DIAGNOSTIC PROCEDURES

unit 20 preparation for procedures

OBJECTIVES

After studying this unit, the student will be able to:

- Identify the steps needed to prepare the patient for a procedure.

- Identify safety precautions needed for any procedure.

- Identify the best way to arrange supplies, equipment, and the room conditions.

- Identify steps in observing and recording.

Some procedures may be carried out by the nurse without direct involvement of another person; testing the urine for sugar and acetone is an example. Other procedures such as the physical examination require the skills of a physician or nurse practitioner. In the physical examination as in almost every diagnostic procedure, the nurse must prepare the patient and gather the equipment needed. The nurse's responsibility is to:

- Follow the doctor's orders promptly and accurately.

- Prepare the patient and the equipment to be used.

- Remain with the female patient throughout the physical exam and during procedures when help is needed.

Procedures vary with different hospitals. However, the principles upon which these procedures are based are widely accepted. In every procedure, provision must be made for the safety and comfort of the patient. The nurse must also consider the economy of time, effort and materials, and the order of the patient unit. Permission of the patient must be obtained to perform all major procedures. The best time to obtain permission is when the treatment is being explained. The

---

Safety Practices with Procedures

- Protect the patient from infection by using good handwashing before and after the procedure.

- Verify the patient's identity by checking the patient's ID arm bracelet before doing the procedure.

- Recheck the doctor's order to avoid errors about the type or time of the procedure.

- Safeguard the patient from falls or injuries which can result from careless transfer methods.

Fig. 20-1 All procedures and treatments require use of safety.

safety of the patient is the responsibility of both the doctor and the nurse.

PSYCHOLOGICAL PREPARATION OF THE PATIENT

The nurse must have a thorough knowledge of the procedure in order to feel secure in performing it and to convey this confidence to the patient. Anxiety, fear or doubt should not be communicated to the patient. Talking with the patient about the procedure may be vital in gaining his confidence.

PROCEDURE

1. Inform the patient when the procedure is to be done. Inform the patient as early as possible.

2. Explain the procedure and urge the patient to ask questions. Use simple words and be sure the patient understands each step.

   The informed patient is more likely to understand the value and purpose of the procedure. This helps gain the patient's cooperation. A common effort may be vital to the success of the procedure.

3. Introduce the patient to the other health team members helping with the procedure.

   This courtesy reduces anxiety and displays a mutual interest in his care.

4. Inform the patient often about the progress throughout the procedure. Allow the patient to signal for needed rest periods during the procedure.

   The patient appreciates even small amounts of control over the pace of the procedure.

PHYSICAL PREPARATION OF THE PATIENT

Proper physical preparation helps give the patient a feeling of confidence. Providing

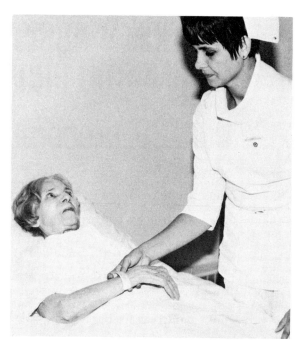

Fig. 20-2 Always check the patient's ID bracelet in preparation for a procedure.

privacy is an important part of the preparation. Screening the patient is required for most procedures. The performance of a procedure may be disturbing to other patients in the room. An awareness of being observed may arouse anxiety in the patient receiving bedside care.

The patient is draped to suit the position necessary for carrying out the procedure. All unnecessary exposure must be avoided. The gown or pajamas should be slack enough to provide adequate working space. The top bedding should be replaced with a drawsheet, being careful not to expose the patient. The top bedding is then fanfolded to the foot of the bed. When needed, a bath blanket should be used for warmth instead of a drawsheet. Examinations can be done easier when the patient wears a hospital gown. Use of a gown also prevents damaging or staining the patient's personal bedclothing.

Many procedures require the patient to assume specific body positions. The nurse should help the patient into the required position if necessary. The patient should not be left in an uncomfortable position for long periods of time. Discomfort will tire and likely irritate the patient.

PREPARATION OF THE ENVIRONMENT

Adequate lighting is essential. This includes general overhead lighting as well as spot lighting. Spot lighting is focused over the specific part of the body involved in the procedure. A gooseneck lamp is usually used for this purpose. The lamp should be set far enough from the patient so it does not cause a burn.

Creating drafts in the room should be avoided. However, good ventilation should be maintained. Good ventilation adds to the comfort of the patient as well as the health team. This, in turn, contributes to the proper performance of the procedure. The room should be in good order before starting a procedure. The surfaces should be cleared and all articles not in use should be put away.

After the procedure all equipment should be washed or taken to the utility room. Supplies should be properly discarded or returned to central supply for cleaning. Soiled sheets, towels and dressings are placed in the laundry.

Chart the type of procedure performed, the time, the person performing it and the observations made.

VOCABULARY

- Define the following words:

acetone	confidence	impersonal
anxiety	gooseneck	psychological

SUGGESTED ACTIVITY

- Set up a role playing situation with another student. Using a few references, study the steps required for a simple procedure such as a dressing change. Explain the procedure to the other student who is acting as a patient. Give the patient a chance to ask questions and be alert to signs which may show doubt or anxiety in the patient.

REVIEW

Select the *best* answer.

1. In every procedure, provision must be made for

    a. the safety and comfort of the patient
    b. economy of time, effort and material
    c. the order and appearance of the unit
    d. all of the above

2. Good handwashing is used

    a. before a procedure only
    b. after a procedure only
    c. before and after a procedure
    d. to sterilize the hands

3. The nurse can be sure of a patient's identity by

   a. asking the patient who he is
   b. checking the patient's ID bracelet
   c. asking other personnel
   d. checking the patient's chart

4. To feel secure about performing a procedure, the nurse should

   a. have a thorough knowledge of the procedure
   b. speak with a physician first
   c. practice the procedure at home
   d. talk about it with other nurses

5. The purpose of explaining the procedure is to

   a. gain the patient's cooperation
   b. help the patient to gain confidence in the physician or nurse
   c. allow the patient to ask questions
   d. all of the above

6. To prepare the patient psychologically for a procedure, the nurse should

   a. check the patient's ID bracelet
   b. introduce the patient to the visitors in the unit
   c. call the social worker
   d. allow the patient to ask questions about the procedure

7. The patient's safety and comfort during a procedure is the responsibility of

   a. the social worker   c. only the nurse
   b. the doctor and nurse   d. only the doctor

8. A hospital gown worn by the patient for a procedure

   a. is sterile
   b. makes the patient more cooperative
   c. makes examining the patient easier
   d. distinguishes one patient from another

9. Proper physical preparation of the patient and the environment

   a. helps give the patient a feeling of confidence
   b. is unimportant
   c. is the responsibility of housekeeping department
   d. excludes screening the unit

10. Preparing the patient's environment includes

    a. maintaining adequate lighting and a 76°F or 24.4°C room temperature
    b. clearing away all the patient's personal articles
    c. maintaining good ventilation
    d. keeping the room dimly lit

unit 21 positioning and draping

OBJECTIVES

After studying this unit, the student will be able to:

- Describe at least three examination positions.
- Name which position is used for circulatory shock.
- Explain how to protect the privacy of a patient during an examination.

Physical examinations can be done in the patient's room or in a specially equipped room. The nurse should see that the lighting and equipment is ready for the procedure being done. Being prepared avoids delays during the procedure.

EXAMINATION POSITIONS

In order to assist with examinations it is necessary for the nurse to know how to position and drape the patient. The type of examination determines the position in which the patient is to be placed. After the

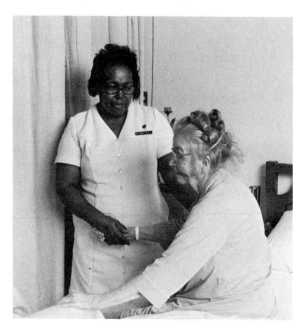

Fig. 21-1 Sometimes an examination can be done in the patient's own room.

procedure is explained, the area should be screened, and the patient given the needed assistance. The body area to be examined is not exposed until the doctor is ready. This adds to the patient's privacy.

Horizontal Recumbent Position

The horizontal recumbent position is one of relaxation and comfort. This position is the one most commonly used for physical examinations. The patient lies flat on the back with legs together, extended or slightly flexed to relax abdominal muscles. If needed, one pillow is allowed under head. The arms may either cross on the chest or lie along the sides of the body.

One drawsheet is spread over the patient and is not tucked in.

Dorsal Recumbent Position

The dorsal recumbent position is used for vaginal and rectal examination. The

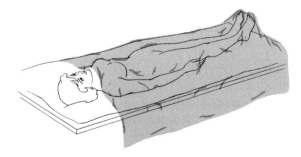

Fig. 21-2 The horizontal recumbent position

91

patient lies flat on the back with knees flexed. One large sheet is spread over the entire body, except the head. The sheet may be drawn back for both vaginal and abdominal examinations. The center of the sheet is folded back to expose the perineum when the physician is ready to examine.

Dorsal Elevated Position

The dorsal elevated position is used for examination of the pelvic organs. This position is the same as the dorsal recumbent position except that extra pillows are placed under the head and shoulders to further relax the abdominal muscles. Draping is the same as for the dorsal recumbent position.

Knee-Chest Position

The knee-chest position, also called the genupectoral position, is used for rectal and vaginal examinations. The patient rests on the chest and knees. The knees are slightly separated with the thighs perpendicular or at a right angle with the bed. The face is turned to one side and may rest on the forearms. Draping is accomplished by use of a large sheet, or by two drawsheets. One drawsheet for the lower part of the body and one for the upper part of the body.

Sims' Position

Sims' position is used for rectal examination and treatments. The patient lies on the left side with the left arm extended behind the back. The body is inclined forward. The legs should be flexed with the right knee drawn up higher then the left. Draping is the same as for the horizontal recumbent position. A portion of the sheet may be folded back to expose the anus or perineum.

Dorsal Lithotomy Position

The dorsal lithotomy position is used for vaginal, rectal and urinary bladder examinations. The patient lies on the back with the buttocks resting on the end of the table. The patient's feet are raised 18 inches above the buttocks and supported in stirrups. Thighs should be at a right angle with the examination table. Knees should be flexed and separated.

Trendelenburg Position

The Trendelenburg position is used for circulatory shock. The patient lies flat on the back with hips and knees elevated. The portion of his legs below the knee rests on an inclined plane slanting downward. Shoulder supports are used to prevent the patient from

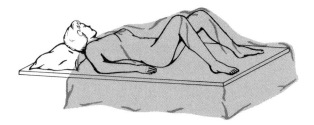

Fig. 21-3 The dorsal recumbent position

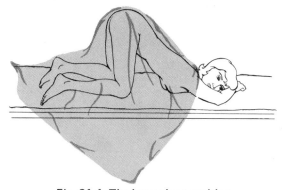

Fig. 21-4 The knee-chest position

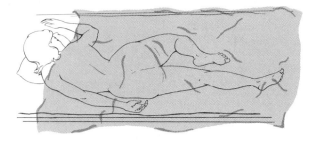

Fig. 21-5 The Sims' position

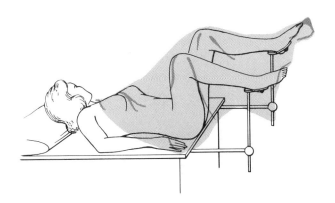

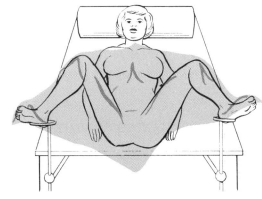

A. The buttocks should rest on the end of the table.

B. The point of the sheet should cover the perineal area.

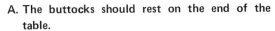

Fig. 21-6 Dorsal lithotomy position

slipping. The treatment will determine the type of draping used.

Upright Position

The upright position is used to observe orthopedic and neurological conditions. The patient stands draped with a sheet passing under the axillae and crossing diagonally over the shoulders and pinned in front. The patient stands in bare feet on a paper towel.

Prone Position

The prone position is used to examine the back or spine. This position is sometimes ordered following back injury or for back surgery. The patient lies on the stomach with the head turned to either side. The patient is draped with one large sheet.

Lateral Position

In the lateral position the patient lies on either side, inclining forward slightly. Draping covers the patient completely up to the neck.

Semi-Fowler's Position

The head of the bed is elevated 45° for the semi-Fowler's position. The trunk of the body should be resting at this 45° angle while lying on the back. No special draping is necessary.

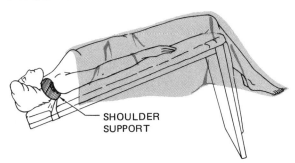

SHOULDER SUPPORT

Fig. 21-7 Trendelenburg position

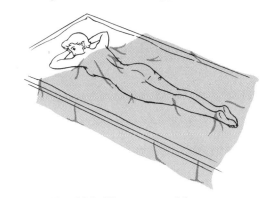

Fig. 21-8 The prone position

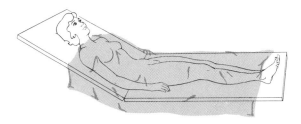

Fig. 21-9 Semi-Fowler's position

VOCABULARY

- Define the following words:

bimanual	lateral	perpendicular
dorsal	lithotomy	prone
genupectoral	perineum	recumbent

SUGGESTED ACTIVITY

- With the help of another student, practice positioning and draping. Determine which positions are the most tiring for the patient.

REVIEW

Briefly answer the following questions.

1. Why is the body area to be examined not exposed until the physician is ready?

2. Name the position which requires the use of stirrups.

3. Which position especially helps abdominal muscles?

4. Name the position which is used for a patient in circulatory shock?

5. What is the name of the position in which the stomach lies flat against the examination table?

unit 22 the physical examination

OBJECTIVES

After studying this unit, the student will be able to:

- Identify equipment needed for a physical examination.
- Describe how to assist the doctor in performing the exam.
- Describe three ways a nurse assists the doctor in performing a physical examination.
- Give two reasons a physical examination may cause uneasiness for the patient.
- List five items a doctor uses in an examination.
- Identify purposes for using three specific examination positions.
- Name which examination follows the vaginal examination.

A doctor performs a physical examination on each patient who is admitted to the hospital. After admission the examination may be repeated to check the patient's progress and to study new symptoms.. A patient may not require a routine physical examination more than once. The nurse should take the time needed to carefully prepare for even brief examinations.

Patients often feel uneasy about having a physical examination. They may fear the outcome or the examination itself. The nurse should be kind and aware of the patient's need for comfort. Knowing how to drape properly gives the patient more privacy. The patient is less embarrassed when the nurse respects this need. Female patients should be attended by a female nurse if the doctor performing the examination is male. The nurse also must assist weak or elderly patients and support them as needed.

Before a routine physical examination, the doctor takes a history. The nurse is often asked to leave until the history has been taken. Patients are usually more at ease answering personal questions when less people are present. The nurse should leave quietly and ask the doctor to call when the history is complete.

PROCEDURE

1. Assemble equipment and take it to the patient's unit or the examination room:

   Emesis basin
   Flashlight
   Hand towel or paper towel
   Lubricant
   Ophthalmoscope (for examining the eyes)
   Otoscope (for examining the ears)
   Percussion hammer (to test reflexes)
   Powdered gloves
   Sphygmomanometer
   Stethoscope
   Tissues
   Tongue depressor
   Laryngeal mirror
   Vaginal speculum (for the female patient)

Equipment may vary. The nurse should know the type of examination to be done and assemble the needed equipment.

The mirror may require special attention. If it is cold, warm, moist breath causes the mirror to fog. (Condensation forms on the mirror.) Placing the mirror in a glass of warm water before the examination prevents this. Be sure the mirror is warmed and dried before the exam.

2. Greet the patient and explain the procedure.

3. Screen the patient's unit, or take the patient to the exam room.

4. Make sure the windows or the ventilation vents do not direct a draft on the patient.

   Prevent chilling the patient.

5. Offer the bedpan or assist the patient to the bathroom.

6. Provide for adequate lighting.

   This will vary according to examination being performed.

7. Lower the treatment table or bed to assist the patient onto it.

   Place the emesis basin nearby.

8. Untie the back of the patient's hospital gown.

9. Introduce the patient to the doctor if they have not already met.

10. Assist the doctor during the examination.

    Pass equipment to the doctor and discard or set aside used articles. When passing the tongue depressor, do not touch either end. This prevents spreading germs into the patient's mouth.

11. Fold top sheet down to the patient's abdomen and loosen the gown for examination of the chest.

12. Assist patient to sit up for posterior chest examination.

    Many patients will need support to remain in the sitting position.

13. Assist the patient to lie down.

14. Fold sheet to the pubic area and raise the gown. Proper draping exposes only the patient's abdomen.

    This prepares the patient for the abdominal examination.

15. Lower the gown and cover the body with the sheet except for the patient's legs.

    Expose both legs at once to permit the doctor to observe the symmetry of the legs.

16. If vaginal examination is to be performed, place patient in dorsal recumbent position and drape her.

    If treatment table is used, lower the foot end and place patient's feet in stirrups. Assist her so that the buttocks rest on the end of the table.

17. Open a package of powdered gloves and assist the doctor in putting them on.

    Sterile technique is used to assist in use of sterile gloves. If nonsterile gloves are used, the nurse should handle them with a towel instead of her hands.

18. Hand the vaginal speculum to the doctor.

    Warm the speculum ahead of time to avoid causing the patient discomfort.

19. Place lubricant on a towel so the doctor can rub the ends of the speculum with the lubricant.

Always use a water base lubricant. (Petroleum jelly which does not dissolve will remain and collect germs around the area.)

20. Set the speculum aside after the doctor is finished with the vaginal examination.

21. Assist the doctor as needed to prepare for the rectal examination.

    While the female patient is in the dorsal recumbent position, the doctor may also perform a rectal examination. For male patients, Sims' position is used. (Females not having a vaginal examination can also be assisted into the Sims' position.)

22. Assist the doctor in putting on sterile gloves.

    Even though the rectum is not a clean area, sterile gloves are usually used.

23. Drop lubricant on a gloved finger.

    Do not touch the glove with the end of the tube or lubricant package.

24. After the doctor has finished examining the patient, tie the patient's hospital gown. If the patient remained in the bed, assist him into a comfortable

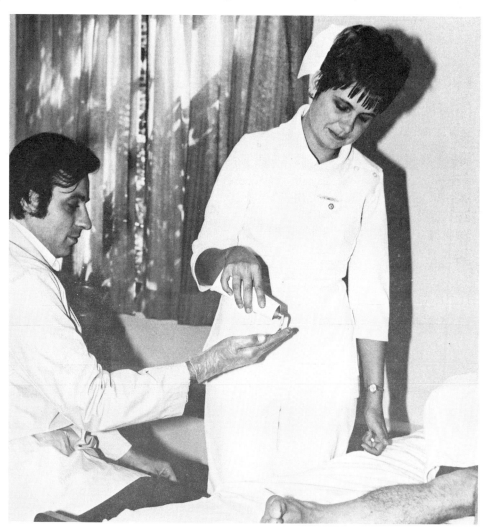

Fig. 22-1 Apply lubricant to the glove without letting the end of the tube touch the glove.

position. If the examination was done in the examination room, assist the patient back to his own room.

Be sure the patient's unit is in order. Place the signal cord within the patient's reach.

25. Clean and replace equipment. Discard used disposable supplies.

26. Record in the patient's chart the name of the doctor who performed the examination. Chart any unusual observations made during the procedure.

VOCABULARY

• Define the following words:

laryngeal	percussion hammer	tongue depressor
ophthalmoscope	posterior	vaginal speculum
otoscope	symmetry	

SUGGESTED ACTIVITY

• Set up a tray in preparation for a routine physical examination. Using a mannequin, practice:

1. Preparation of the patient
2. Draping and positioning the patient
3. Anticipating the physician's needs

REVIEW

Briefly answer the following questions.

1. What is the nurse usually expected to do while the physician obtains the history from the patient?

2. Name two reasons why a physical examination may cause the patient to feel uneasy.

3. List four pieces of special equipment a doctor uses for performing a physical examination.

4. For a female patient, which area is usually examined immediately after the vaginal examination?

5. Why should the nurse avoid touching the end of the tongue depressor when passing it to the doctor?

6. What position does the patient assume for a posterior chest exam?

7. What instrument is used for the vaginal examination?

8. Which position allows the doctor to check the rectum on a male?

9. When is a female nurse usually required to remain with the doctor and the patient?

10. Why are both legs observed at once?

unit 23 height and weight measurements

OBJECTIVES

After studying this unit, the student will be able to:

- Identify one reason for obtaining an accurate weight.

- Determine the appropriate time at which to use the metric system.

- Identify one condition which may cause rapid weight gain.

- Identify two units of measurement used in the metric system.

- Identify one step taken before assisting the patient onto the scale.

The patient's height and weight are required on admission, or as part of a physical examination. Weight alone is often recorded daily. This shows important changes which may occur during the hospital stay. For instance, rapid weight gain may occur with edema. Knowing the correct weight of a patient is also important for the doctor in prescribing certain medications.

A patient who cannot stand on an ordinary scale will need a bed scale or a portable chair scale. Each hospital has different equipment for weighing these patients. Bed scales require the patient to be lifted off the bed. The patient can be spared some effort if the nurses change the linen while the patient is being weighed.

Use of the metric system is increasing in patient care. Measuring height and weight in metric for both infants and adults is becoming more common. The nurse should be familiar with the metric system. The tables in figure 23-2, page 102, provide equivalent measures of pounds with kilograms, and inches with centimeters. Daily use of the metric system provides the best method of learning.

PROCEDURE

1. Check the balance scale for accuracy.

   Before putting the patient on the scale, set the weights on zero. If the pointed end of the balance bar is centered so that it does not touch the guide, the scale is balanced.

2. Place a paper towel on the scale platform.

   This protects patients from possible infection. The paper provides for cleanliness, since many people step on the scale platform in street shoes.

3. Have the patient remove his robe and slippers before stepping on the scale.

   The patient should be wearing about the same amount of clothing each time he is weighed.

4. Move the large weight to the number which measures about fifty pounds under the patient's weight.

   For most adults, this weight rests on the 100 or 150 mark.

Desirable Weights for Men and Women Twenty-Five and Over: Weight in Pounds According to Frame, in Indoor Clothing

MEN

Height (with shoes on) 1-inch heels		Small Frame	Medium Frame	Large Frame
Feet	Inches			
5	2	112-120	118-129	126-141
5	3	115-123	121-133	129-144
5	4	118-126	124-136	132-148
5	5	121-129	127-139	135-152
5	6	124-133	130-143	138-156
5	7	128-137	134-147	142-161
5	8	132-141	138-152	147-166
5	9	136-145	142-156	151-170
5	10	140-150	146-160	155-174
5	11	144-154	150-165	159-179
6	0	148-158	154-170	164-184
6	1	152-162	158-175	168-189
6	2	156-167	162-180	173-194
6	3	160-171	167-185	178-199
6	4	164-175	172-190	182-204

WOMEN

Height (with shoes on) 2-inch heels		Small Frame	Medium Frame	Large Frame
Feet	Inches			
4	10	92-98	96-107	104-119
4	11	94-101	98-110	106-122
5	0	96-104	101-113	109-125
5	1	99-107	104-116	112-128
5	2	102-110	107-119	115-131
5	3	105-113	110-122	118-134
5	4	108-116	113-126	121-138
5	5	111-119	116-130	125-142
5	6	114-123	120-135	129-146
5	7	118-127	124-139	133-150
5	8	122-131	128-143	137-154
5	9	126-135	132-147	141-158
5	10	130-140	136-151	145-163
5	11	134-144	140-155	149-168
6	0	138-148	144-159	153-173

(For women between 18 and 25, subtract 1 pound for each year under 25.)

Fig. 23-1 Knowing average heights and weights for adults helps in evaluating a patient's measurements.

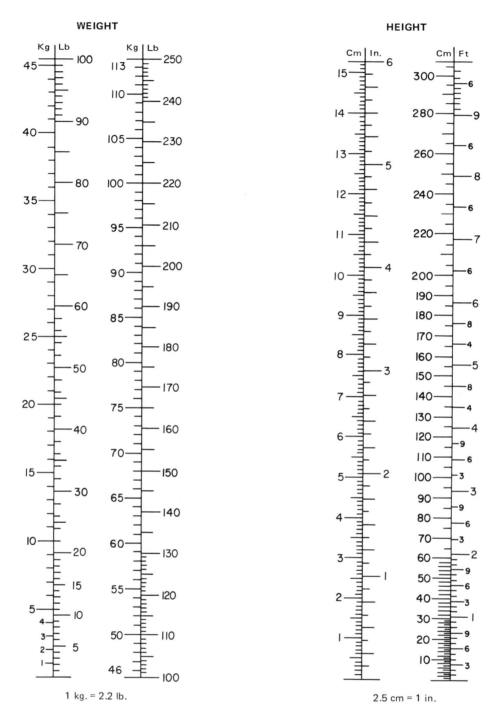

Fig. 23-2 Metric conversion scales for weight and height

5. Move the small weight indicator to the left until the bar balances in the center of the guide.

6. Add the number under the small weight indicator to the large number under the other indicator. Record the patient's weight in the chart.

7. Convert pounds to kilograms if hospital policy requires use of the metric system.

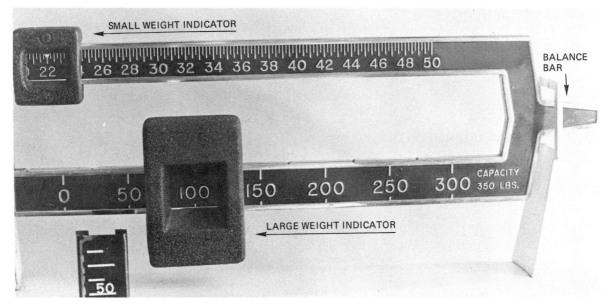

Fig. 23-3 The correct weight is obtained when the balance bar is centered in the guide.

Change pounds to kilograms by dividing the weight in pounds by 2.2 (2.2 pounds equals one kilogram.) For example a weight in pounds is 122. 122 ÷ 2.2 = 55.8 kilograms.

8. While the patient is still standing on the scale, instruct him to stand erect.

   Feet should be at the center of the scale platform.

9. Raise the height scale rod so the top is above the head. Move the bar of the height scale down until the bar rests flat on the patient's head.

   The bar should rest at a right angle, or perpendicular to the height rod.

10. Read the scale and record the height in the chart.

    Convert inches to feet and inches. For example, a scale which reads 67 inches can be divided by 12 since 12 inches equals one foot. A height of 67 inches converts to 5 foot 7 inches.

11. Convert the inches to centimeters if hospital policy requires use of the metric system.

    To convert inches to centimeters, multiply the number of inches by 2.54 (2.54 centimeters equals one inch.) A height of 5'7" = 67 inches. 67 inches x 2.54 = 170 centimeters.

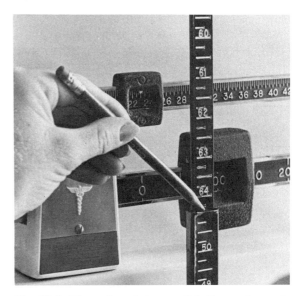

Fig. 23-4 The point of the pencil indicates the mark from which the height is read.

VOCABULARY

- Define the following words:

  average   portable

  conversion   scale

SUGGESTED ACTIVITIES

- Practice balancing the scale.

- Weigh and measure members of the class. Compare with standards given in figure 23-1.

- Practice converting inches to centimeters and pounds to kilograms. Use the formulas below to check the values given in the tables in figure 23-2.

$$1 \text{ kg} = 2.2 \text{ lb.}$$
$$2.54 = 1 \text{ in.}$$

REVIEW

Select the *best* answer.

1. A condition which may cause rapid weight gain is
   a. dehydration   c. scales
   b. edema   d. infection

2. Accurate weight information is essential for doctors who are
   a. prescribing certain medications
   b. planning the patient's discharge
   c. testing equipment
   d. studying the metric system

3. Two units of measure in the metric system are
   a. pounds and kilograms   c. centimeters and inches
   b. pounds and inches   d. kilograms and centimeters

4. Before the patient steps on the scale, the nurse should
   a. place a paper towel on the platform
   b. ask the patient to remove robe and slippers
   c. balance the scale
   d. all of the above

5. The nurse should record height and weight using the metric system when
   a. the doctor requests it
   b. the nurse becomes familiar with it
   c. hospital policy instructs the nurse to do so
   d. state law requires it

unit 24 collection of specimens: urine

OBJECTIVES

After studying this unit, the student will be able to:

- List the laboratory tests done in a urinalysis.
- Identify steps used for obtaining a routine urine specimen.
- Explain the procedure for collecting a 24-hour urine specimen.

A routine urine specimen is collected for a test called a *urinalysis*. A urinalysis is the most common laboratory test performed. The complete test includes a study of color and degree of cloudiness; pH, which shows an acid or alkaline reaction; specific gravity, which measures its concentration; tests for glucose and protein (albumin). Microscopic examination in addition shows the presence of blood, pus or *casts*. Casts consist of a gel usually made up of dead cells.

A specimen of urine is routinely sent to the laboratory on the admission of the patient. Before surgery a urinalysis is required. At other times, the early morning specimen is usually used. The doctor usually specifies the time to collect the specimen.

COLLECTING SPECIMENS

The nurse should check to see that specimens are collected correctly. The outside of the container must not be contaminated with the specimen. This protects those who handle the specimens. The nurse should also be sure of the doctor's order. Confusion with an assignment causes delay and extra effort for the staff and the patient. Tests which must be repeated may lengthen the patient's hospital stay. This is costly and unnecessary. The nurse should understand the tests which are ordered and know how to prepare for them. Patients have more confidence in a nurse who understands the steps of procedures being performed.

LABELING

An important part in collecting specimens is completing the label correctly. The label should include.

- Patient's full name
- Patient's hospital or case number
- Room number and bed
- Physician's name
- Date and time of collection
- Type of examination needed

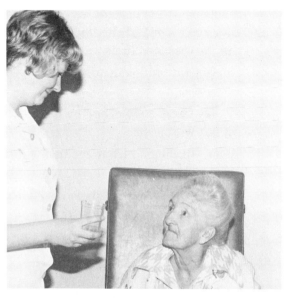

Fig. 24-1 Understanding the purpose of the urine test ordered reduces error in collecting the specimen.

The addressograph can be used on some labels. The date and time of collection and type of test should not be omitted, however. Most specimens are sent to the lab with a laboratory slip. The slip gives the details about the test ordered. The doctor's order should be checked before preparing the label. *All unlabeled specimens should be discarded.*

ROUTINE URINE SPECIMEN

The routine urine specimen or urinalysis should be prepared carefully. Procedures which are routine require as much attention as those which are ordered special.

PROCEDURE

1. Assemble supplies:
   Label
   Laboratory requisition slip properly filled out
   Bedpan or urinal and cover
   Container and cover for specimen
   Graduate pitcher

2. Greet the patient and explain the procedure.

   Try not to embarrass the patient in explaining the procedure. Focus on the importance of the test rather than on the specimen itself.

3. Screen the unit and offer the bedpan or urinal.

   Toilet tissue should not be discarded in pan with urine.

4. Pour specimen from bedpan into graduate.

   Record the amount if patient's intake and output is to be measured.

5. Pour about 120 ml (4 oz.) into the specimen container.

6. Wash the hands.

   Do not contaminate outside of container.

7. Cover container. Attach label and requisition slip to container. Include the information required by hospital policy.

   Use the labeling guidelines presented earlier in this unit.

8. Clean and replace equipment according to hospital policy.

9. Take or send specimen to laboratory.

   Report any unusual observations immediately to supervising nurse.

10. Record:

    Time of specimen collection
    Type of specimen (Routine urine specimen or urinalysis)
    Amount collected
    Any unusual observations

THE 24-HOUR URINE SPECIMEN

The doctor may request a patient's urine to be collected for a 24-hour period. A 24-hour specimen which is *quantitative*, consists of the total urine volume collected in one specimen. (In another type of specimen, the 24-hour urine will be divided and collected in three parts. The doctor will specify the time for each of the three urine collection periods.) All types of 24-hour specimens should remain on ice. Some urine tests require a chemical to be added to the container to preserve the specimen. The nurse should check the laboratory procedure manual before preparing these specimens.

PROCEDURE

1. Assemble supplies:

   1 gallon 24-hour urine collection bottle, labeled (disposable or nondisposable)
   Laboratory requisition slip
   Bedpan or urinal
   Graduate pitcher

Label should include: type of 24-hour specimen, patient's full name, patient's room and bed number, patient's hospital number, date of collection, time started.

2. Greet the patient and explain the procedure.

Be sure the patient understands that each specimen must be collected and kept in the bottle. Lost urine should be reported immediately since this may require the patient to begin a new 24-hour specimen.

3. At the starting time, have the patient void. Discard this urine.

This assures that the specimen contains only urine produced within the specified 24 hours. The patient begins the 24-hour period with an empty bladder.

4. Collect all urine the patient voids for 24 hours and put it in the labeled bottle.

The specimen should not be contaminated with feces. Dependable patients may be taught to collect their own specimen.

5. At the end of the 24-hour period, have the patient void and add this urine to the bottle also.

Be sure of the starting time. Careful records are needed since different nurses will be responsible for collecting the specimen within the 24-hour period.

6. Cover the specimen and wash the hands.

Do not contaminate the outside of the container.

7. Record the following information on the laboratory slip, the collection bottle, and in the patient's chart:

Type of 24-hour specimen
Time started
Total volume of specimen
Amount sent to laboratory (if different from total)

8. Attach the requisition slip and the label.

9. Send the entire amount of the urine collected to the lab unless the doctor's order specifies otherwise.

At times the doctor will ask the nurse to mix the specimen well and then send

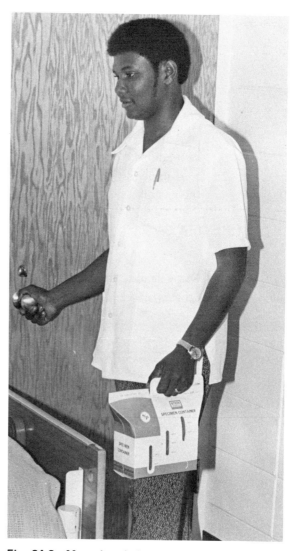

Fig. 24-2 Many hospitals now use a disposable 24-hour urine container.

only 120 ml (4 oz.) to the lab. The doctor may ask that the specimen be sent in three parts as mentioned earlier.

10. Clean and replace equipment according to hospital policy.

VOCABULARY

- Define the following words.

acid	feces	pus
albumin	fraction	quantitative
alkaline	glucose	specific gravity
casts	microscopic	specimen
concentration	pH	urinalysis

SUGGESTED ACTIVITIES

- Using outside sources, study the following 24-hour urine tests and identify which conditions or diseases may be diagnosed as a result of the tests.

  a. Albumin (quantitative)

  b. Addis count

  c. Catecholamines

- Ask another student to role play as a patient. Assume the patient is dependable and ambulatory and explain the procedure for collecting a 24-hour urine. Be sure the patient understands by having him repeat the instructions.

REVIEW

A. Briefly answer the following questions.

1. Name three places information is recorded when collecting a 24-hour urine specimen.

2. What should be done with a specimen which is unlabeled?

3. a. Should the urine voided at the beginning of the 24-hour period be collected for the 24-hour specimen?

b. Should the urine voided at the end of the 24-hour period be collected?

4. What should the nurse do if part of a 24-hour urine specimen is lost?

5. Name two occasions when the urinalysis is done routinely.

B.   List the tests performed in a urinalysis.

unit 25 testing urine for sugar and acetone

OBJECTIVES

After studying this unit, the student will be able to:

- State the normal level of blood sugar in the body.
- Identify and explain the tests used for checking sugar in the urine.
- Identify and explain the tests used for checking acetone in the urine.

Testing urine for sugar and acetone is usually the nurse's responsibility. Since the tests are simple to do, these specimens are not sent to the laboratory. The procedure is ordered daily and in some cases four times a day, before meals and at bedtime. Tests for sugar and acetone help the doctor determine the condition of the patient. The results provide a guide for prescribing treatments.

DIABETES

Tests for sugar and acetone are most commonly ordered for diabetic patients. In diabetes, the islets of Langerhans in the pancreas do not produce enough insulin to use up or oxidize sugar. Therefore, insulin or a similar drug is given to maintain the normal level of sugar in the blood. The normal blood sugar level is 60-90 mg per 100 ml. When the blood sugar levels exceeds 170 mg per 100 ml, sugar can be detected in the urine. Testing the urine for sugar tells the doctor how much insulin is being used by the body. The tests, therefore, help the doctor determine the dosage of insulin required by the patient. The tests also help the doctor regulate the patient's sugar intake through a prescribed diet. This is done with the schedule, selection and portions of food prescribed.

The simple sugar for which the urine is tested is called *glucose*. The presence of glucose in the urine is called *glycosuria*. When an excessive amount builds up in the urine, *hyperglycosuria* occurs. The normal amount of glucose in the urine cannot be detected with the routine test used.

An examination of the urine specimen should indicate the most recent changes in the blood sugar level. The patient should void one-half hour before the time the specimen is to be taken. This urine is discarded since it may have been in the bladder for a few hours. The urine collected for the specimen then is fresh and provides the most accurate picture of the body's need for insulin.

Among the tests available which are used to detect sugar in the urine are the Clinitest tablets, Tes-Tape paper strips, and dipsticks which have treated squares placed along a plastic strip. These three methods are simple and fast to use. The Benedict test also detects sugar in the urine. However, this test requires a heating device and therefore is not convenient to use. Directions for using the tablets or strips are printed on the bottle labels. The instructions should be followed carefully to obtain good results. Most products have an expiration date printed on the label as well. The testing materials should be used within that stated period of time only.

TESTING FOR SUGAR: Clinitest Tablets

Clinitest tablets provide a fast, easy method for testing urine for sugar. The tablets produce colors which clearly identify the amount of sugar in the urine. The nurse should remember not to touch the tablets and to keep the container tightly closed.

PROCEDURE

1. Assemble equipment:

    Urine in specimen container
    Test tube
    Medicine dropper
    Clinitest tablet
    Water
    Clinitest color chart

2. Place 5 drops of urine in test tube with medicine dropper.

    Test tube must be clean and dry. Hold medicine dropper upright so that urine does not touch the sides of the test tube.

3. Rinse medicine dropper in cold water. Add 10 drops of water to test tube with dropper.

    Hold medicine dropper upright.

4. Remove Clinitest tablet from the bottle by dropping the tablet into the bottle cover. Cover the bottle tightly.

    CAUTION: Do not touch the tablet with the fingers. Burns can occur if the tablet contacts moisture on the hand.

5. From the bottle cover, drop the tablet into the test tube. Watch reaction carefully. Fifteen seconds after the reaction has stopped, shake test tube gently. Compare resulting color with color chart.

    Do not handle the test tube during the reaction since it becomes hot. Time the waiting period with second hand of watch. Use Clinitest color

chart. The final color and the speed of the reaction depend upon the level of sugar. A specimen which turns orange can be recorded 2% or 4+.

─────Color Changes Indicating Sugar─────	
0%	Blue (normal)
1/4% – 1/2%	Green (trace to +)
3/4% – 1%	Tan (++ to +++)
2%	Orange (++++)
over 2%	Dark greenish brown

6. Discard the urine from the test tube.

7. Clean and replace equipment according to hospital policy.

    Drain test tube in test tube rack.

TESTING FOR SUGAR: Tes-Tape

Tes-Tape is narrow light-colored paper which is made in rolls. The container looks

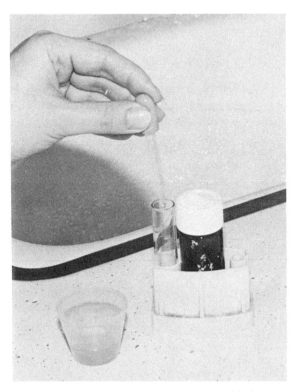

Fig. 25-1 Drops of urine and water are added to the test tube before the Clinitest tablet.

like a Scotch tape holder. The paper is treated to react to the presence of glucose in urine.

PROCEDURE

1. Assemble equipment on tray:

   Urine in specimen container
   Container with Tes-Tape

2. Lift lid and pull out about 4 cm (1½ inches) of tape.

3. Close lid and tear off the tape by pulling straight out.

   Do not touch the end of tape which will be placed in the urine. Moisture from the hands may alter the test results.

4. Dip 0.6 cm (1/4 inch) of the tape into the urine container and remove it immediately.

   The end of the tape held between the fingers should be kept dry.

5. Hold the tape out of the urine for one minute before reading the results.

   If urine is free of glucose, the color of the tape remains unchanged.

6. Compare tape with the color chart on the outside of the container.

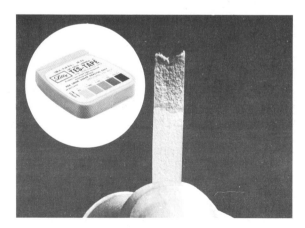

Fig. 25-2 After being dipped in the specimen, the Tes-Tape is compared with a color chart.

7. Record the time, test results, and any unusual observations.

   Report any unusual reaction to the charge nurse as soon as possible.

TESTING FOR SUGAR: Dipsticks

The dipstick is a plastic strip which has one or more treated squares at one end. Some dipsticks have as many as six different testing squares. The testing square for glucose can be located by reading the label on the container of the dipsticks.

PROCEDURE

1. Assemble equipment:

   Urine in specimen container
   Container with dipsticks

2. Remove one dipstick from the container.

3. Close container tightly.

   Humidity can ruin the testing squares.

4. Completely immerse the testing squares on the strip in the urine for 2 seconds.

5. Tap the edge of strip against the urine container to remove excess urine.

6. In exactly 30 seconds compare the test square with the color chart provided on the bottle.

7. Record the time, test results, and any unusual observations.

   Report any unusual reaction to the charge nurse as soon as possible.

TESTING FOR ACETONE

Testing the urine for acetone is usually ordered with tests for suger. Sometimes patients do not take in enough carbohydrates or cannot use carbohydrates properly. As a result, they use fats for energy instead of carbohydrates. The patient may not be eating well or may be under stress. This could occur with overexercise, illness, or a problem with body functions. The test for acetone indicates the presence of ketone bodies in the urine. Ketones, which result from fat breakdown, act as poisons to the body when they remain in the blood stream. Acetone in the urine indicates an important change in the body which requires the doctor's attention.

TESTING FOR ACETONE: Acetest Tablets

Using Acetest tablets indicates the amount of acetone present in the urine. These tablets often are kept in a kit with the bottle of Clinitest tablets. The Acetest almost always follows a test for sugar.

PROCEDURE

1. Assemble equipment:

   Urine specimen
   Bottle with Acetest tablets
   Dry white paper
   Medicine dropper

2. Remove one Acetest tablet from the bottle by shaking it into the cap. Then, without handling the tablet with the fingers, place it on plain white dry paper.

3. Place only 1 drop of urine on the acetest tablet with a medicine dropper.

   One drop should be enough urine to moisten the tablet.

4. Wait 30 seconds. Compare resulting color with color chart.

5. Discard the tablet into the toilet and flush it. Discard paper and the rest of the urine.

   Never leave tablets or medicines where patients or visitors could handle them.

6. Clean and replace equipment according to hospital policy.

7. Record the time, test results and any unusual observations.

   Report any unusual observations to the supervising nurse.

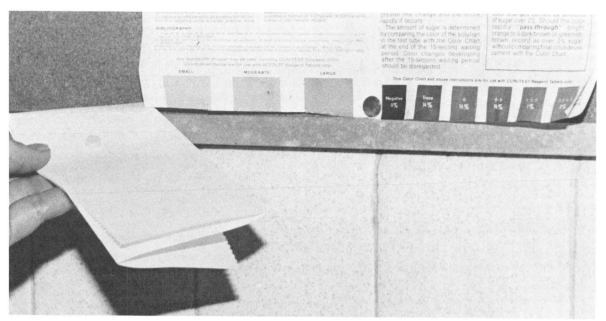

Fig. 25-3 Acetest tablets change from light pink to various shades of purple.

TESTING FOR ACETONE: Dipsticks

Dipsticks for detecting acetone are like those used for glucose. Often the glucose and acetone testing squares appear together on the same dipstick. The nurse should read the label on the container to locate the square which tests acetone. Three brand names for the dipsticks used are Ketostix, Keto-Diastix or Multistix. The nurse should become familiar with the method of testing used in the particular hospital.

PROCEDURE

1. Assemble equipment:

    Bottle containing the dipsticks
    Urine in container
    Color chart provided with product

2. Remove one dipstick from the container.

3. Close the container again tightly.

4. Dip the testing squares into the urine and hold for two seconds.

5. Gently tap edge of strip against the urine container.

6. After exactly 15 seconds, compare the test square with the color chart.

7. Record the time, test results, and any unusual observations.

Report any unusual results to the charge nurse.

VOCABULARY

- Define the following words:

acetone	glycosuria	medicine dropper
carbohydrates	hyperglycosuria	oxidize
diabetes	insulin	pancreas
dosage	islets of Langerhans	reaction
expiration date	ketone bodies	

SUGGESTED ACTIVITIES

- If laboratory facilities are available, use whatever urine test is available and test your own urine for sugar and acetone using the correct procedure for that method.

- Obtain the liquids below and test them for sugar:

    unsweetened orange juice
    tomato juice
    water

REVIEW

A. Briefly answer the following questions.

1. Why is testing the urine of the diabetic patient so important?

2. Why should the patient void one-half hour before the designated time for testing the urine for sugar?

3. If urine tests for sugar are ordered q.i.d., at what times are they done?

4. Give the normal level of blood sugar in the body.

5. How can the nurse avoid touching the Clinitest and Acetest tablets with the fingers?

B. Match the term in Column II with the correct description in Column I.

Column I

_____ 1. tablet which tests for sugar
_____ 2. technical term for sugar in the urine
_____ 3. equivalent to 2% or the orange colored urine
_____ 4. plastic strip having testing squares at one end
_____ 5. secrete insulin in the body
_____ 6. products of fat breakdown
_____ 7. requires one drop of urine for one tablet
_____ 8. method of regulating sugar intake
_____ 9. a simple sugar
_____ 10. indicates that tablets are no longer usable

Column II

a. glycosuria
b. ketone bodies
c. dipstick
d. Acetest
e. Clinitest
f. islets of Langerhans
g. diet
h. expiration date
i. 4+
j. glucose
k. 2+
l. protein in the urine
m. gland which secretes glucose

unit 26 collection of specimens: stool

OBJECTIVES

After studying this unit, the student will be able to:

- List four types of stool specimen collection.
- Identify one step important in each of the four types of stool collection.
- Determine the correct way to warm a specimen.
- Identify three reasons for using good handwashing.

A specimen of stool is a sample of fecal material collected in a special container to be sent to the laboratory for examination. The laboratory report aids the physician in making a diagnosis. The label attached to the container must show the patient's identification and the examination to be done. The nurse should check the doctor's order to be sure the correct exam will be shown on the label. The most common types of tests are for disease-producing microorganisms, parasites, occult blood and chemical analysis.

TYPES OF STOOL SPECIMENS

Collection for Cultures

Bacteria or viruses are both microorganisms which may be found in the stool. In order to be detected, they must grow and multiply in the stool. This requires the laboratory to prepare a culture of the stool. The stool is sent to the lab as soon as it is collected. If a delay cannot be avoided, the specimen must be kept cold or frozen. Only a small amount is needed. The specimen may be collected with a large cotton swab and be placed in a sterile test tube to be sent to the lab. Using a sterile test tube is essential. A sterile tube contains no organisms. Therefore, if organisms are found in the specimen examination it is safe to conclude they

were not in the test tube before the specimen was added.

Collection for Parasites

A *parasite* is an organism which lives on or within another organism. The parasite depends on the other and takes food and energy away from the other organism. Some worms, flukes and protozoa are parasites to the human. When stool is to be examined for parasites, it must be kept at body temperature and examined within 30 minutes. If the doctor has determined that the organisms are in the active state, the entire stool must be collected for a specimen and sent to the laboratory.

Collection for Occult Blood

Occult blood is blood which is hidden, in this case in the stool. Blood becomes dark after it passes through the body and is hard to detect. A patient who is bleeding inside often excretes blood through the stool. A specimen for occult blood need not be examined immediately or be kept warm. A meat-free diet may be ordered preceding this examination because meat residue may give a false report.

Collection for Chemical Analyses

Chemical analyses may be performed for a great number of reasons. For this test the entire day's elimination must be collected. If there is more than one stool in the 24-hour period, all should be sent. Usually the specimen is kept cold if there is a delay between collection and examination.

PROCEDURE

1. Assemble equipment:

    Bedpan and cover
    Label
    Specimen container and cover
    Toilet tissue
    Tongue blades

    Label should include: Examination to be done, patient's full name, patient's room number, patient's hospital number, date and time of collection.

2. Explain to the patient that a stool specimen is needed and that a bedpan must be used. Give the patient a warm bedpan if the type of specimen requires it.

    If possible, allow the patient to provide a specimen from the daily bowel movement.

3. Take the bedpan and the specimen to the utility room.

4. Use tongue blades to remove the specimen from the bedpan. Place the specimen in the container.

    The amount required depends on the examination to be done.

5. Wash the hands thoroughly.

    Do not contaminate the outside of the container.

6. Cover the container and attach a completed label.

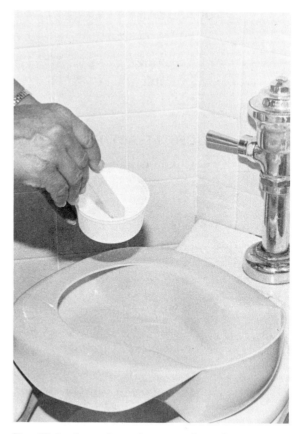

Fig. 26-1 A stool specimen can be collected easily from the patient's bedpan.

Make sure the cover fits over the container tightly. If the specimen should be kept warm, place the container on top of a hot water bag.

7. Clean and replace the equipment according to hospital policy.

8. Take or send the specimen to the laboratory promptly.

9. Record in the chart:

    Time
    Type of examination ordered
    Observations: Color, consistency and odor

    Report any unusual observations immediately to the supervising nurse.

VOCABULARY

- Define the following words:

culture	parasite	stool
occult	sterile	virus
organism		

SUGGESTED ACTIVITY

- Obtain permission to visit the laboratory of a local hospital. If possible, observe the incubation of stool culture in process.

REVIEW

A.   Select the *best* answer.

1.   The nurse can determine whether occult blood is in a stool specimen by

   a. looking for bright red streaks in the stool
   b. sending the specimen to the lab for examination
   c. asking the patient if he has been bleeding
   d. asking for the opinion of the doctor

2.   A specimen to be examined for parasites needs to be

   a. kept warm and examined within 30 minutes of collection
   b. kept cold or frozen
   c. free of meat residue
   d. sent for a culture

3.   A stool specimen is kept warm by

   a. keeping it in a low temperature oven
   b. placing it in an open container
   c. leaving it in a dry warmed bedpan
   d. placing it on a hot water bag

4.   The nurse should wash the hands before putting a cover on the specimen container to

   a. prevent contaminating other nurses
   b. prevent spreading disease to lab personnel
   c. avoid contaminating the outside of the container
   d. all of the above

5.   Stool which is to be examined for cultures is placed in a sterile test tube to

   a. keep the specimen sterile
   b. protect personnel from disease spread
   c. prevent other organisms from entering the specimen
   d. grow and multiply better

B.   List four types of stool specimen collections.

unit 27 collection of specimens: sputum

OBJECTIVES

After studying this unit, the student will be able to:

- Name two sources of sputum in the body.
- List the characteristics of sputum which should be observed and recorded.
- Indicate the quantity of sputum desired for a specimen.
- Identify the definition of bronchi.
- Explain three steps in a sputum collection procedure.
- Name two diseases detected by sputum examination.
- Name three terms used to describe sputum quantity.

A sputum specimen aids the doctor in diagnosing problems in the respiratory system. *Sputum* is a mucous substance expelled by clearing the throat or by coughing. This matter may come from the lungs or *bronchi*, the tubes entering the lungs. Sputum may consists of a discharge from the nasal or throat area. Depending on the patient's disease, sputum may consist of pus, blood, mucus and microorganisms. Sputum is profuse in some diseases. Remember that the nurse observes symptoms but does not diagnose the medical condition.

It is important for the nurse to observe the sputum when collecting it and to chart the observations accurately. The amount of sputum, the appearance (consistency and color), and the odor are significant.

- Amount: The amount may be scant, moderate, or copious (plentiful).
- Appearance: Sputum containing pus may be yellow, gray or black. A rusty color or streaks of red blood may indicate pneumonia. An abscess in the lungs may create a green-colored sputum.
- Odor: The odor may be described as sweet, putrid (foul).

A sterile specimen container is used for collecting sputum. This assures that the lab will identify only organisms from the specimen and not from some other source. One bacterium which may be present in the sputum is the tubercle bacilli. This type of bacterium causes pulmonary tuberculosis. The pneumococci, which is a circular bacteria, is the cause of pneumonia. Many other bacteria and viruses can multiply in the sputum and cause disease.

The patient should be instructed to cough deeply in order to bring up material from the bronchi and lungs. Otherwise, the specimen consists only of saliva and nose and mouth secretions. The specimen may be collected at any time the patient is able to produce the sputum. Sometimes a 24-hour collection of sputum may be ordered. Other times only one specimen may be needed.

PROCEDURE

1. Assemble equipment:

   Container for the specimen
   Glass of water
   Tissues
   Emesis basin
   Label

   Label should include: Patient's full name, type of examination, patient's room number, patient's hospital number and date and time of collection.

2. Greet patient and explain the procedure. Screen the unit.

3. Have patient rinse mouth.

   This removes food particles. Use an emesis basin for waste.

4. Ask patient to cough deeply to bring up sputum and expectorate into container.

   Have the patient cover his mouth with a tissue to prevent spread of infection.

5. Collect 15-30 ml (1-2 tablespoons) of sputum unless otherwise ordered.

6. Wash the hands.

   Avoid contaminating the outside of the container.

7. Cover the sputum container and attach the label.

   Be sure the label is filled out properly.

8. Clean and replace equipment according to hospital policy.

9. Take or send the specimen to the laboratory promptly.

   Avoid allowing the specimen to become dry.

10. Record:

    Date and time
    Specimen of sputum sent to laboratory
    Observations: Color, consistency, odor.

    Report any unusual observations immediately to supervising nurse.

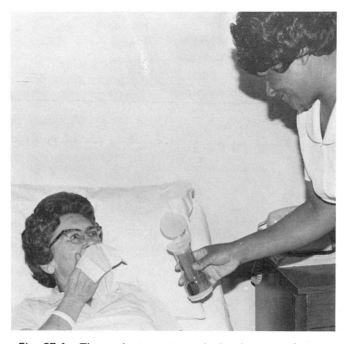

Fig. 27-1 The patient must cough deeply to produce a sputum specimen.

VOCABULARY

- Define the following words:

abscess	expectorate	pulmonary tuberculosis
bronchi	foul	putrid
consistency	mucus	scant
copious	pneumococci	sputum
expel	pneumonia	tubercle bacilli

SUGGESTED ACTIVITY

- Discuss with the instructor the ways used to help a patient produce sputum for a specimen. Consider using the help of a respiratory technician and the equipment.

REVIEW

Briefly answer the following questions.

1. Name two sources of sputum in the body.

2. Identify the name of the breathing tubes which enter the lungs.

3. What three important characteristics of sputum should the nurse observe and record?

4. What condition may rusty color or blood-streaked sputum indicate?

5. What amount of sputum is usually collected for a specimen?

6. Why should the patient cover his mouth while coughing?

7. What three terms are used to describe the amount of sputum produced?

8. Why should the nurse assist the patient to cough deeply?

9. Name the diseases caused by these two bacteria:

    a. tubercle bacilli

    b. pneumococci

10. Why is the patient instructed to rinse the mouth before producing a sputum sample?

unit 28 collection of specimens: vomitus

OBJECTIVES

After studying this unit, the student will be able to:

- Identify the characteristics of vomitus which should be observed and recorded.

- Differentiate projectile vomiting from regurgitation.

- Identify the proper way to handle an emesis basin which contains a specimen.

The doctor may request a specimen to be taken in the event that a patient vomits. The nurse should save the vomitus in a covered emesis basin and call it to the attention of the doctor. To assist the patient, support the head and turn it to the side. Hold the emesis basin against the face to catch the vomitus. Wipe the patient's mouth with a tissue and allow the patient to rinse with water. Do not give water to a postsurgical patient if the doctor has prohibited it. See that the patient is comfortable before preparing the specimen.

Label the basin with the patient's name. The doctor may or may not order a specimen to be sent to the laboratory. If he orders a specimen to be sent, the nurse prepares the label with the essential information. The nurse then attaches it to the specimen container and takes or sends it to the laboratory for examination.

When a patient vomits, it is necessary for the nurse to report the following characteristics of the specimen:

- Color: green or greenish yellow (bile); bright red (fresh blood); "coffee grounds" or reddish brown (digested blood)

- Presence of foreign matter such as pus, mucus, feces, blood or undigested food.

- Manner in which the patient vomited. Vomiting with great force, usually with little warning, is called *projectile vomiting*. Vomiting with little or no force is called *regurgitation*.

VOCABULARY

- Define the following words:

  bile
  digested

  projectile vomiting
  regurgitation

SUGGESTED ACTIVITY

- Discuss why vomiting is often expected of patients returning from surgery.

REVIEW

Select the *best* answer.

1. Vomitus which contains digested blood appears

   a. bright red
   b. green

   c. like coffee grounds
   d. milky

2. Vomitus which contains bile

   a. is odorless
   b. appears green or greenish yellow
   c. appears reddish brown
   d. should be discarded immediately

3. Projectile vomiting is that which

   a. requires little or no effort
   b. contains mucus
   c. is regurgitated
   d. is expelled with great force

4. Foreign matter in the vomitus includes

   a. pus
   b. feces

   c. blood
   d. all of the above

5. The emesis basin containing the specimen should be

   a. labeled
   b. burned after use
   c. kept in the utility room
   d. left uncovered until the doctor sees it

unit 29 assisting with venipuncture

OBJECTIVES

After studying this unit, the student will be able to:

- Determine the definition and purpose of a venipuncture.
- List five types of tests that are performed on blood specimens.
- Determine which health personnel are permitted to start an I.V.
- Describe steps in the procedure used to perform a venipuncture.
- Describe steps in the procedure used to start an I.V.

The introduction of a hollow needle into a vein is called *venipuncture*. It is performed to take blood for a specimen or to give intravenous infusions. To obtain a specimen, the median cubital vein or its branch, the median basilic vein, are used most frequently. Both of these veins are in the forearm. The veins of the back of the hand may be used. Occasionally, a specimen of blood is drawn from veins of the leg or foot. Doctor's orders will specify if a period of fasting is to precede the test.

In many hospitals a laboratory technician performs this procedure and brings the necessary equipment. However, in other hospitals a nurse or doctor performs the venipuncture. In this case the nurse will set up the necessary equipment. For blood tests, different colored test tubes are used for the various tests. The nurse should be sure the correct tubes are provided. Blood tests are valuable diagnostic tools. The types of blood examinations are too many to list. The general groups, however, can be listed as follows:

- blood cell studies
- biochemical tests
- hormone levels
- antibody and blood grouping studies
- tests for microorganisms

The venipuncture is also performed to give intravenous infusions, (I.V.). The I.V. supplies fluids through the veins when the patient cannot take fluids by mouth. An I.V. may be used to give the patient a special drug.

When an intravenous infusion is ordered, the doctor sets the rate of flow. The condition of the patient, the type of solution, and the amount of fluid to be given determine the rate of flow. The maximum rate of flow is set by the size of the needle chosen. Adjusting the pinch clamp or the height of the bottle affects the rate of flow. The nurse must make sure that the rate of flow is maintained as the doctor ordered it.

Subcutaneous edema is swelling just under the skin. This occurs if the rate of flow is too high or if the needle becomes dislodged. Edema which is not corrected can lead to shock.

OBTAINING A BLOOD SPECIMEN

The nurse is responsible for seeing that ordered blood tests are obtained. Care should be taken to see that the correct test is done soon after it is ordered. Orders which are overlooked or errors which are made cause extra effort for both the patient and the staff.

PROCEDURE

1. Assemble equipment:

   Alcohol swabs
   Small emesis basin
   Adhesive strips
   Requisition slip properly filled out
   Labeled test tube
   2 No. 19 or 20 needles
   Sterile hypodermic syringe
   Tourniquet

   Label should include: Examination to be done, patient's full name, patient's room number, patient's hospital number, date and time.

2. Greet patient and explain the procedure.

3. Screen the unit.

4. Introduce the person taking the specimen to the patient if they have not already met.

5. Raise the sleeve to the patient's upper arm.

6. Provide a tourniquet for the doctor, nurse or technician to apply.

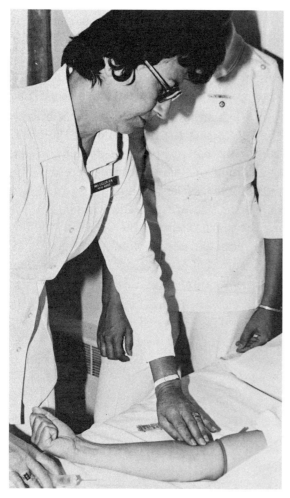

(A) Applying a tourniquet and asking the patient to make a fist helps blood to collect so the vein can be located.

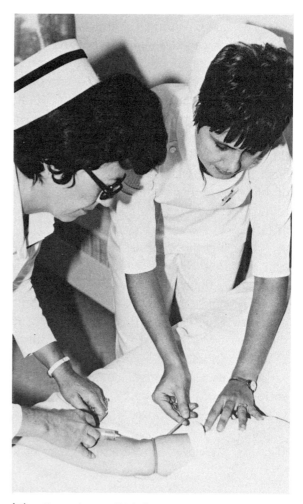

(B) Once the needle is inserted releasing the tourniquet allows blood to be withdrawn into the syringe.

Fig. 29-1 Assisting with a venipuncture.

7. Provide alcohol swabs to clean the venipuncture area.

8. Provide a syringe and needle with a protective cover.

9. Release the tourniquet if requested to do so, once the needle is inserted and blood appears in the syringe.

   If no blood appears in the syringe, another venipuncture may be necessary.

10. Place the test tubes within easy reach of the person performing the venipuncture.

    Be sure the test tubes are the correct color for the tests being done. Also be sure they are properly labeled.

11. After the needle is withdrawn, hold a cotton ball moistened with alcohol over the venipuncture site.

    Patients who are alert can do this themselves.

12. When the bleeding has stopped, place a temporary Band-Aid over the site.

    This applies pressure to the area and keeps the area clean.

13. Wash the syringe and needle in cold water immediately if they are not disposable.

    This prevents blood from clotting and plugging the needle and syringe.

14. Discard disposable equipment. Clean and replace other materials according to hospital policy.

15. Record in the patient's chart the time, type of tests to be done on the blood specimen and any observations.

16. Take or send the specimen to the laboratory.

STARTING AN INTRAVENOUS INFUSION

The therapy provided by an I.V. may be the most important aspect of a patient's care. Nourishment and drugs can be given through the I.V. Fluid replacement is all that is required for some patients. An I.V. is usually started by a doctor or a registered nurse. Many hospitals now have special I.V. teams which start I.V.s and take blood specimens throughout the hospital. The nurse assisting others with starting an I.V. must learn the steps used. This makes the procedure progress faster and more smoothly.

PROCEDURE

1. Assemble equipment:

   Alcohol swabs
   Cotton balls
   Small emesis basin
   Adhesive tape
   Standard sterile I.V. infusion set, tubing and drip chamber
   Armboard
   I.V. solution as ordered
   Needles and catheters of various types and sizes
   Tourniquet
   2 x 2 gauze squares
   Band-Aids
   I.V. pole or stand

2. Explain the procedure to the patient. Ask the patient to remain still when the needle is inserted.

   Explaining the procedure helps the patient relax and cooperate better.

3. Screen the unit and provide good lighting.

4. Set out the needed equipment within easy reach.

5. Cut strips of adhesive tape about four inches long and hang them from the supply tray.

6. To assist the person starting the I.V., have the tourniquet and sponge ready when needed.

7. Check to see that the solution and tubing is connected and hangs properly from the pole.

   This is usually set up by a person trained in the I.V. procedure.

8. Hand the desired needle or catheter to the person starting the I.V.

9. Uncover the end of the I.V. tubing without touching the tubing.

   The end of tubing connects to the needle and must remain sterile.

10. Assist in holding the patient still if needed.

11. Release the tourniquet when ordered and have tape and gauze ready to secure the needle in the arm.

12. Assist in applying the armboard to the patient's arm.

    The armboard restricts motion so the needle does not dislodge.

13. Discard disposable supplies and clean other equipment properly.

14. Record the date, time, amount and type of solution; I.V. site, name and status of person who started the I.V.; any unusual observations noted during the procedure.

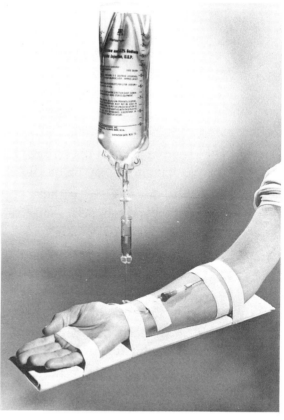

Fig. 29-2 For I.V. infusions an armboard helps secure the needle in place.

VOCABULARY

- Define the following words:

antibody	hormonal	subcutaneous
basilic	hypodermic	tourniquet
biochemical	infusion	venipuncture
fluid replacement	median cubital	

SUGGESTED ACTIVITIES

- Arrange to visit a local hospital. If possible, observe a lab technician draw a blood specimen in the laboratory or in the outpatient department. Check the procedure used with the one described in this unit. Have the technician explain the steps being used.

- If laboratory facilities are available, ask the instructor to assist you in setting up the equipment needed for an I.V. infusion. Observe the different types of needles and catheters used as well as the containers and tubing for the solutions.

REVIEW

A. Briefly answer the following questions.

1. For what purpose is a venipuncture performed?

2. For a blood specimen or an I.V., how is the site prepared before the needle is inserted?

3. Which veins are used most often for drawing a blood specimen?

4. Name five types of examinations which can be done with a blood specimen.

5. Why is a nondisposable needle and syringe washed with cold water after being used?

B. Select the *best* answer.

1. The person who decides on the rate of flow for an I.V. infusion is the
    a. doctor
    b. registered nurse
    c. I.V. technician
    d. practical nurse

2. Swelling around the venipuncture site which occurs from escaped fluid is called

   a. ascites
   b. displacement
   c. subcutaneous edema
   d. shock

3. Three persons who in most facilities would be starting an I.V. are the

   a. aide, the practical nurse or the registered nurse
   b. practical nurse, the I.V. technician or the registered nurse
   c. doctor, the charge nurse, or the pharmacist
   d. doctor, the registered nurse or the I.V. technician

4. A piece of equipment which is to remain sterile and therefore should not be touched with the fingers is the

   a. end of the I.V. tubing
   b. armboard
   c. I.V. solution bag
   d. tourniquet

5. Venipuncture is defined as

   a. the infusion of fluids into the vein
   b. the introduction of a hollow needle into a vein
   c. the withdrawal of blood from the vein
   d. a subcutaneous swelling

unit 30 assisting with gastric intubation

OBJECTIVES

After studying this unit, the student will be able to:

- Describe four methods of determining whether the nasogastric tube is in the stomach.
- Give two purposes of performing a gastric intubation.
- Explain the steps used in performing a gastric intubation.
- Explain why gastric contents are examined.

Examination of gastric contents can reveal the concentration of the secretions and the presence of blood, pus, or microorganisms. To reach the stomach, a tube must pass from the nose, through the esophagus and into the stomach. The tube is therefore called a *nasogastric tube* (N-G tube) and the process, *intubation*. Gastric intubation is usually performed by a doctor but may be done by a nurse who is taught to do it. The nurse should understand the steps of the procedure whether or not she actually performs it.

Gastric intubation is required for reasons other than obtaining specimens. Sometimes patients are fed through a nasogastric tube. The contents of the stomach may need emptying before surgery. Swallowed poisons or stomach distention may create a need to empty the stomach. A suction machine is often used to empty the stomach in these cases. To withdraw a specimen, however, usually the suction created by a syringe is sufficient.

PASSING THE TUBE INTO THE STOMACH

The nasogastric tube is passed through the nose. Passing the tube through the mouth can be done but it causes more gagging and discomfort. After passing through the nose, the N-G tube should enter the esophagus.

However, the tube can enter the trachea instead. This can block the patient's air passage in addition to causing discomfort. The nurse must watch the patient for signs of dyspnea and cyanosis. The N-G tube may also fail to enter the esophagus if it rolls up in the back of the throat. Various methods have been devised to determine when the N-G tube enters the stomach. The person performing the procedure is likely to choose one of the following methods.

- Ask the patient to hum. If the tube is close to the larynx, the patient is unable to hum. This indicates the tube should be withdrawn and reinserted.
- Insert the free end of the N-G tube into a glass of water. If air bubbles appear in the water, the tube is in the trachea and must be removed at once.
- Insert air into the free end of the N-G tube using a syringe. A stethoscope is placed over the stomach region. If a swoosh of air is heard with the stethoscope, the tube is in the stomach.
- Withdraw air from the N-G tube using a syringe. If the tube is in the stomach, greenish yellow fluid can be withdrawn from the tube.

PROCEDURE

1. Assemble equipment:

   - Gastric tube (N-G tube)
     Water-soluble lubricant
     Glass of ice water and drinking tube
     Tissue wipes
     Emesis basin
     Rubber or plastic sheet
     Cotton drawsheet
     Bulb syringe or 20 ml syringe
   - Polyethylene tubes are preferred. They are more comfortable for the patient. If a rubber tube is used, it must be placed in a basin of ice to make it firm and easy to pass.

2. Greet the patient and explain the procedure if the doctor has not already done so.

   The procedure should be explained before the equipment is brought to the bedside.

3. Screen the unit.

4. Raise the head of the bed so that the patient is in semi-Fowler's position. If the patient cannot tolerate this position, the dorsal recumbent position may be used.

5. Drape patient's shoulders with a waterproof sheet. Cover the waterproof sheet with a cotton drawsheet.

   This procedure may cause the patient to gag or regurgitate.

6. Pick up the perforated end of the tube about 15 cm (6 inches) from the tip and lubricate it about 10 cm (4 inches).

   Normal saline solution may be sufficient as a lubricant. The doctor will state a preference. Oil-based lubricant is not used because it could possibly cause infection if it should be aspirated into the lung.

7. The doctor or nurse holds the tube so that it droops. In this drooping position, the tube is inserted into the patient's nostril.

8. Ask the patient to flex his neck so that the chin rests on the chest. Ask him to swallow and encourage mouth breathing. If sips of water are permitted, this may make the passage of the tube less difficult.

   Flexion of the neck makes it easier for the patient to swallow. This flexed position smooths the curve of the pharyngeal wall and helps prevent the

A
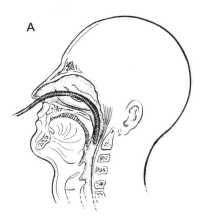

B
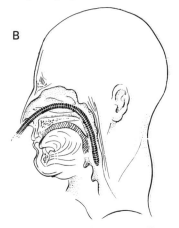

Fig. 30-1 Flexing the neck allows the N-G tube to pass through more easily.

tube from entering the trachea. The doctor passes the tube a few inches with each swallow. Peristalsis helps to move the tube along, and deep breathing minimizes gagging. The doctor may not give the patient sips of water because water dilutes the specimen.

9. When the tube is thought to be in the stomach, the nurse assists with one of the tests listed on page 131 to confirm the location of the tube.

   The person performing the procedure decides which method is best to test the location of the tube.

10. Detach the syringe and empty its contents into the specimen container.

11. Place the syringe in the emesis basin.

12. If the doctor orders the tube to be removed, pinch the N-G tube at patient's nostril. Withdraw it so that no fluid can drip from it as it passes the trachea. **NOTE:** The nurse should not remove an N-G tube unless she has been taught to do this procedure.

Have a small towel ready to receive the tube. Withdraw the tube quickly and smoothly.

13. Wash the patient's hands and face and provide mouthwash.

14. Replace soiled linen as necessary.

15. Adjust the bed for the patient's comfort.

16. Clean and replace all equipment according to hospital policy.

17. Take or send the specimen to the laboratory.

18. Record:

    Procedure: Gastric Intubation
    Name of doctor or nurse who
      performed the procedure
    Observations: color, consistency,
      unusual material
    Condition of the patient

VOCABULARY

- Define the following words:

distention	larynx	pharyngeal
gastric	nasogastric	syringe
intubation	peristalsis	trachea

SUGGESTED ACTIVITIES

- Obtain a chart of the human body showing a side view of the internal organs of the head and torso. Trace the pathway taken by a nasogastric tube from the nose to the stomach. Notice the body structures which might cause resistance as the tube is passed.

- Conduct the following experiment using a paper straw and a glass of water. Draw the water into the straw with suction from your mouth. While the water is in the straw and you continue to apply suction, pinch the straw and remove it from the water. Describe what happens. Does the water remain in the straw, or does it drip out? Conduct the same experiment, except do not pinch the straw before withdrawing it from the water. Describe the results. Explain how the results of these experiments are similar to withdrawing a nasogastric tube.

REVIEW

Briefly answer the following questions.

1. Who usually performs a gastric intubation?

2. What can be determined by examining gastric contents?

3. For what purposes, other than obtaining a specimen for analysis, may gastric intubation be performed?

4. Why should an emesis basin be included with the other equipment needed for this procedure?

5. Using the test with the glass of water, what indicates that the tube is in the trachea?

6. Why is the tube passed through the nose rather than the mouth?

7. Why must the tube be pinched before it is withdrawn?

8. Explain why the doctor in some cases does not allow the patient to take sips of water for easing passage of the tube?

9. Describe how the test using the syringe and stethoscope determines when the N-G tube has passed into the stomach.

10. Why is the patient asked to flex the neck while the tube is being passed?

unit 31 assisting with a lumbar puncture

OBJECTIVES

After studying this unit, the student will be able to:

- Name four purposes of performing a lumbar puncture.
- Name the examinations done on a specimen of spinal fluid.
- Explain steps used to assist with the lumbar puncture.
- Describe what is meant by aseptic procedure.
- Describe the appearance of normal spinal fluid.

A *lumbar puncture* is the insertion of a hollow needle into the spinal canal between the third and fourth lumbar vertebrae for the purpose of withdrawing fluid. The procedure may be performed for one of the following reasons:

1. To obtain a specimen for examination to determine the presence of blood or microorganisms
2. To withdraw fluid to relieve pressure
3. To inject dye before a myelogram or to inject air for a pneumoencephalogram
4. To measure the pressure of the spinal fluid
5. To administer a spinal anesthetic

A lumbar puncture is an *aseptic* procedure. This means that the puncture site must be free from germs and that sterile equipment is used. The nurse should also explain the procedure to the patient. This greatly affects the success of the procedure. Part of the nurse's duty is to assist the doctor and to prevent contaminating the gloves, equipment and skin area. In addition, the nurse must see that the patient remains in the required position. The nurse holds the patient in the curved position to keep the patient still, figure 31-1.

PROCEDURE

1. A tray with *all equipment sterilized* is sent from central supply. It contains the following items:

   Drape with a central opening
   Towels
   Hypodermic needle and syringe
   Ampule of anesthetic
   Spinal needles with stylets
   Extra syringe and medication if ordered
   3-way stopcock and manometer
   Test tubes
   Sterile dressing and adhesive tape

   When the lumbar puncture set is commercially prepared and entirely disposable, the following items are included. In most sets, they are the only items which are needed in addition to the sterile tray pack:

   Sterile gloves
   Forceps
   Antiseptic solution for skin preparation
   3" x 3" sponges to apply antiseptic to puncture site

2. Greet the patient and explain the procedure.

Stress the importance of remaining still throughout the procedure.

3. Place the patient at the side edge of the bed.

4. Arch the patient's back by flexing the head toward the chest and flexing the knees toward the chin. Move the shoulders forward.

   This position widens the space between the vertebrae making the insertion of the needle easier. The nurse must assist the patient in maintaining this position without movement. Throughout the procedure which follows, the nurse notes carefully the reaction of the patient, and any changes in color, pulse, and respiration.

5. The doctor sets up a sterile field. To do this the doctor puts on gloves, paints the puncture site with antiseptic solution, and drapes the area.

6. The doctor injects the antiseptic and then inserts the lumbar puncture needle.

   As soon as the fluid begins to drip, he attaches the manometer to measure pressure. Taking the spinal fluid pressure is usually part of the procedure for obtaining a specimen.

7. When the manometer has been removed, the doctor fills the specimen tubes as the fluid drips from the needle.

   Normally, spinal fluid is clear and colorless.

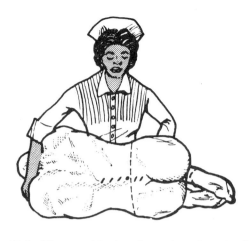

Fig. 31-1 When positioning the patient for a lumbar puncture, flex the head and the knees so the back is rounded.

8. After the doctor withdraws the needle, a sterile dressing is applied to the puncture site.

   The nurse should be sure enough sterile dressings are provided.

9. Make the patient comfortable and ask the patient to lie flat in bed for the time the doctor specifies.

   The doctor may request the patient to lie flat for 12 to 24 hours. This helps prevent headaches.

10. Clean and replace equipment according to hospital policy.

11. Label the test tubes containing the specimens.

12. Record in the patient's chart:

    Date
    Time
    Name of the doctor who performed
        the procedure
    Purpose of the lumbar puncture
    Observations made about the patient

VOCABULARY

- Define the following words:

ampule	aseptic	manometer
anesthetic	lumbar	myelogram

pneumoencephalogram	spinal canal	stylet
puncture	stopcock (3-way)	vertebrae
sterile field		

SUGGESTED ACTIVITIES

- Working with another student, take turns placing each other in a position for a lumbar puncture.

- Set up the equipment for a lumbar puncture. Assume the equipment is sterile.

REVIEW

A.   Name four purposes of performing a lumbar puncture.

B.   Briefly answer the following questions.

1.   What is meant by aseptic procedure?

2.   Describe the appearance of normal spinal fluid.

3.   What three nursing duties are required for a lumbar puncture?

4.   Why is the patient's back curved for this procedure?

5.   What examinations are done on a specimen of spinal fluid?

SELF-EVALUATION V

A. Match the facts in column I with the related terms in column II.

Column I   Column II

_____ 1. position in which patient   a. gastric intubation
          sits at 45° angle to bed   b. tourniquet
_____ 2. test for sugar in urine   c. lubricant
_____ 3. used for a vaginal   d. Trendelenburg
          examination   position
_____ 4. appearance of digested   e. speculum
          blood   f. projectile vomiting
_____ 5. position used for circula-   g. parasites
          tory shock   h. bile
_____ 6. colors vomitus yellow green   i. bronchi
_____ 7. structure in the respiratory   j. sputum
          tract   k. aspiration
_____ 8. medium which may contain   l. regurgitation
          tubercle bacillus   m. acetone
_____ 9. vomiting with little effort   n. Clinitest
_____ 10. passing a tube into the   o. semi-Fowler's position
          stomach   p. "coffee-grounds"
_____ 11. vomiting with great force   q. Sims' position
_____ 12. jelly which reduces friction r. expectoration
_____ 13. substance in urine which   s. viruses
          shows fat breakdown
_____ 14. equipment used in perform-
          ing a venipuncture
_____ 15. position for a rectal
          examination

B. Complete each sentence by putting the correct word in the blank space
   or spaces.

1. For vaginal examination the patient is placed in _____
   position.

2. The health team member who makes the diagnosis is the _____.

3. The most common laboratory examination is the _____.

4. In order to protect any person who handles a specimen, care must be
   taken not to contaminate _____.

5. To collect a 24-hour specimen, the first voiding is _____
   and the last voiding is _____.

6. Another name for the genupectoral position is _____.

7. Dressing a patient in a _____ facilitates examination.

8. Certain examinations done on blood require the patient to _____ for a period preceding the drawing of the blood.

9. The nondisposable needle and syringe used for venipuncture must be flushed immediately after use to avoid _____ the needle and syringe.

10. During a physical examination both legs should be exposed at once in order to observe _____.

11. The time recommended for collecting a single specimen of urine is _____.

12. The nurse should assist the patient to sit up straight for the _____ examination.

13. To ease insertion, a vaginal speculum should be _____ before it is used.

14. The instrument used to examine the eyes is the _____.

15. The veins in the _____ are usually used for venipuncture.

C. Select the *best* answer.

1. Any unusual observation which the nurse notes while collecting a specimen should first be

   a. charted for the physician's information
   b. reported to the nearest physician
   c. reported to the supervising nurse
   d. told immediately to the patient

2. When handling a specimen for laboratory examination, the nurse should wash the hands

   a. one-half hour before and after caring for the patient
   b. only after covering the specimen container
   c. before covering the specimen container
   d. before entering the utility room

3. The part of the body to be examined by the physician is usually exposed

   a. by the nurse just before the physician is ready to examine the area
   b. by the physician before beginning the examination
   c. just after the patient unit has been screened
   d. by the patient at the physician's request

4. The nurse usually leaves the examination room

    a. when the physician examines the genital organs
    b. during the entire examination
    c. during the taking of the patient's history
    d. none of the above

5. Rapid weight change may be expected if the patient

    a. is scheduled for surgery   c. is overweight
    b. has cancer   d. has edema

6. If the stool is to be collected for occult blood, the patient is placed on

    a. a meat-free diet   c. NPO for 8 hours
    b. a salt-free diet   d. a soft diet

7. If the stool is to be collected for a culture, it must be

    a. kept warm in case of delay in examination
    b. kept cold or frozen in case of delay
    c. collected over a 24-hour period
    d. none of the above

8. A sputum specimen must be sent to the laboratory immediately

    a. to prevent the specimen from drying
    b. to enable examination for blood
    c. so that the color and odor may be detected by the laboratory technician
    d. none of the above

9. Characteristics of a vomitus specimen which should be reported by the nurse are

    a. amount, color and consistency
    b. color, foreign matter and manner of vomiting
    c. amount, foreign matter and manner of vomiting
    d. color, amount and manner of vomiting

10. The following tests are used for detecting the presence of sugar in urine.

    a. Benedict and acetone   c. Clinitest and Wasserman
    b. Clinitest and Guthrie   d. Benedict and Clinitest

11. In order to pinpoint the time of sugar spillover into the urine,

    a. warm the specimen
    b. use the early morning specimen
    c. discard the first specimen; obtain another in a half hour
    d. test urine after meals

12. To collect a sputum specimen correctly, the nurse should
    a. keep the specimen warm
    b. use a sterile container
    c. ask the patient to rinse his mouth with antiseptic solution before producing a specimen
    d. collect the specimen after a meal

13. In diabetes the islets of Langerhans do not produce enough insulin to
    a. oxidize proteins   c. break down fats
    b. oxidize sugar   d. store glycogen

14. The introduction of a hollow needle into a vein is called
    a. intravenous infusion   c. venous pressure
    b. hypodermodipis   d. venipuncture

15. When a specimen of blood is drawn for examination,
    a. veins in leg or foot are most commonly used
    b. a tourniquet is usually not necessary
    c. a doctor's order will specify if fasting is to precede the test
    d. wash the needle in hot water if it is not the disposable type

16. In diabetic patients, ketone bodies increase as a result of
    a. unoxidized sugar   c. lack of exercise
    b. rapid breakdown of fats   d. undigested food

17. The testing method which may determine the presence of both ketones and sugar in urine is called the
    a. dipstick   c. Tes-Tape
    b. Clinitest   d. Acetest

18. The position of the back for a lumbar puncture is
    a. straight   c. hyperextended
    b. curved   d. twisted

19. Aseptic technique is used for a
    a. gastric intubation   c. lumbar puncture
    b. physical examination   d. nonsterile procedure

20. Swelling around a venipuncture site occurs most commonly with
    a. an I.V. infusion   c. a lumbar puncture
    b. obtaining a blood specimen d. a vaginal examination

21. When explaining a procedure to the patient, the nurse should
    a. discourage the patient from asking too many questions
    b. let the patient do all the talking
    c. use simple words
    d. insist that the patient cooperate

22. Physical preparation of a patient for a procedure includes all except
    a. screening the unit
    b. draping the patient
    c. observing for signs of anxiety
    d. dressing the patient in a hospital gown

23. The position used for a gastric intubation is
    a. Trendelenburg
    b. Sims'
    c. knee-chest
    d. semi-Fowler's

24. A sputum specimen is observed for
    a. color, scantness and viscosity
    b. amount, appearance and odor
    c. origin, consistency and the manner expelled
    d. blood, pus and feces

25. Insulin is produced in the
    a. pancreas
    b. liver
    c. fatty tissue
    d. kidney

SECTION VI MAINTAINING THE PATIENT'S SAFETY AND COMFORT

unit 32 turning the patient in bed

OBJECTIVES

After studying this unit, the student will be able to:

- List three hazards of extended bedrest.
- Describe the steps used to assist a patient in changing positions.
- Name two devices which promote comfort and good alignment in bed patients.

Turning a patient is essential for the patient's safety and comfort. The patient who requires bedrest often cannot move or turn easily. The nurse must help the patient change positions in order to help prevent the hazards of bedrest. Some of these hazards are:

- Loss of muscle tone — Lack of exercise causes a muscle to lose its strength and its normal tension.
- Muscle contracture — Poor posture in bed causes muscles to shorten and become stiff.
- Decubiti — Prolonged pressure over one skin area cuts off the blood supply. Skin which does not receive enough oxygen and nutrients, breaks down quickly. This forms an open sore which is difficult to heal.

The nurse can minimize these hazards. No matter how correct or comfortable a position is, the patient must be turned every hour. Patients who can turn themselves should be encouraged to do so. Frequent turning improves general circulation as well as preventing the hazards of bedrest. Muscles receive more exercise if the patient exerts most of the effort. This also spares the patient the sense of helplessness which results from having to wait for the nurse to assist.

TURNING THE PATIENT TOWARD THE NURSE

Whenever possible, turning the patient toward the nurse is preferable. To protect both the patient and the nurse, use of good body mechanics is needed. The help of other team members should be requested when necessary.

PROCEDURE

1. Greet the patient and explain how the turning will be done.
2. Stand close to the patient with one foot in front of the other and the knees bent.

   One knee should brace the nurse's body against the side of the bed.

3. Place one hand on the patient's shoulder and the other on the hips.
4. Roll the patient toward you, slowly and gently.
5. Go to the other side of the bed.

6. Place hands under the patient's hips and pull the patient toward the center of the bed.

   If patient's head and shoulders have also been shifted toward the edge of the bed, place hands under shoulders and move toward the nurse.

7. Place the patient's body in good alignment.

   Use pillows to support the patient if necessary.

TURNING THE PATIENT AWAY FROM THE NURSE

Turning the patient away from the nurse is only done when turning toward the nurse is too difficult. This may occur when room equipment or room activities allow better access to one side of the bed. The nurse should be careful not to push the patient. A rolling action helps protect both the nurse and the patient from injury.

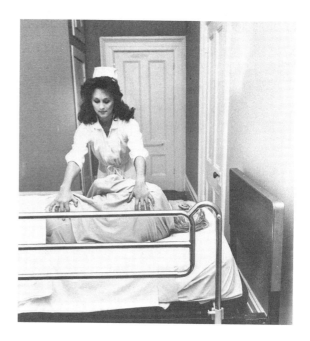

Fig. 32-1 Whenever possible, turn the patient toward you rather than away.

PROCEDURE

1. Greet the patient and explain the procedure.

2. Raise the siderail on the side of the bed to which the patient will be turning.

3. While the patient is lying on his back, have the patient flex his knees. Cross his arms over his chest.

4. The nurse should place one hand beneath the patient's shoulders and the other under the small of his back. **Gently pull the patient to the near side of the bed.**

5. Place your forearms under the patient's hips and move them to the near side of bed.

6. Move patient's ankles and knees to the near side of the bed by placing one

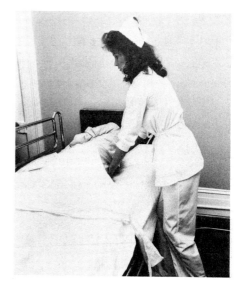

Fig. 32-2 Gently roll the patient away rather than pushing the patient.

   hand under the ankles and one hand under the knees.

7. Cross the patient's nearer leg over the other leg at the ankles.

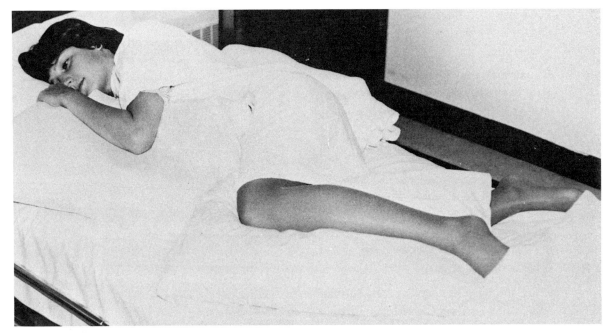

Fig. 32-3 Lying in Sims' position is very comfortable for the patient.

Remember the patient's knees are still flexed and the patient is lying on the back.

8. Roll the patient away from you, slowly and carefully.

Patient is lying on the side.

9. Place hands under the patient's shoulders and draw the patient back toward the center of the bed.

10. Place hands under the patient's hips and move hips to the center of the bed.

Make sure that the patient's body is in good alignment.

MAKING THE PATIENT COMFORTABLE

After changing the patient's position, the nurse should leave the patient in comfort. Providing correct posture and comfort is an important part of a patient's care. The Sims' position is used when the patient lies on the side. Pillows support the arm, leg, head and back. Health facilities which cannot provide this many pillows suggest the use of rolled

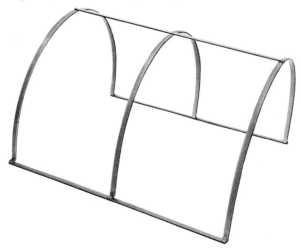

Fig. 32-4   A bed cradle lifts the bedcovers off the patient's legs.

towels or blankets. The nurse should use the materials available and give the patient the best care possible.

Bed Cradle

A device used to maintain the patient's comfort is the bed cradle. It prevents the weight of the bedding from resting on some part of the body. For special uses, the cradle is placed over fractered limbs, burns and skin lesions. Bedding can be placed inside the cradle for warmth and comfort if needed.

Footboard

The footboard or footrest is a device placed between the feet and the end of the bed to maintain the feet at right angles to the legs. It is used to prevent footdrop. *Footdrop* is a muscle contracture which occurs from poor foot and leg alignment in bed. Even a period of three weeks in bed may cause a degree of footdrop. This makes walking difficult when the patient becomes well enough to get out of bed.

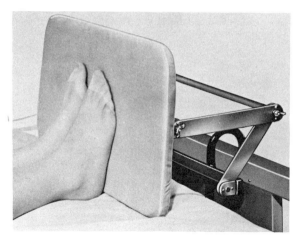

Fig. 32-5 Supporting the feet with a footboard keeps the legs in alignment.

VOCABULARY

- Define the following words:

| brace | decubiti | hazard |
| contracture | footdrop | nutrients |

SUGGESTED ACTIVITIES

- Working in groups, practice moving and turning. Students should evaluate each other's skill in using good posture and good body mechanics.
- Study and discuss with the instructor the hazards of bedrest. Consider the following topics:
    1. Use of range of motion exercises for muscle tone.
    2. Use of lumbar pad, heel support, trochanter roll, finger roll and pillows to preserve body alignment.
    3. Prevention and treatment used for decubiti.

REVIEW

Briefly answer the following questions.

1. Give two reasons the nurse should encourage the patient to change positions with as little help as possible.

2. How frequently should a helpless patient be assisted in a change of position?

3. List three hazards of extended bedrest.

4. Why should the patient be moved toward the nurse whenever possible rather than away from her?

5. Name two devices which add to the patient's comfort and help promote good alignment.

unit 33 moving the patient up in bed

OBJECTIVES

After studying this unit, the student will be able to:

- Identify steps in the procedure used to move a patient up in bed.
- Identify at least one application of good body mechanics.

Patients who are weak or elderly slide down in the bed easily. Hospital beds are usually elevated at the head. Even when the patient is supported by pillows, slipping down toward the foot of the bed occurs. This position is not comfortable and promotes poor posture. Therefore, one or two nurses should assist a patient out of the slumped position.

PROCEDURE

1. Explain procedure.

   Encourage the patient to cooperate and help as much as possible.

2. Lock the wheels of the bed.

3. Lower the head of the bed and remove all pillows.

   This lowers the resistance to moving up.

4. Have patient flex the knees and brace the feet firmly on the bed.

   Assist in flexing the knees and place the feet if necessary.

5. Stand with one foot forward; bend the knees and brace one knee against the bed.

   Putting one foot ahead of the other provides a broader base of support. Toes should be pointed toward the head of the bed.

6. Place one arm under the patient's shoulders. Place the other arm under the back.

Cradle patient's head in bend of your elbow.

7. Face the head of the bed. Slide patient toward the head of the bed, shifting your weight from the rear leg to the forward leg.

   If patient is able to help, on a given signal have the patient push against mattress with both feet.

8. Obtain the assistance of another nurse if the patient is heavy or cannot tolerate movement.

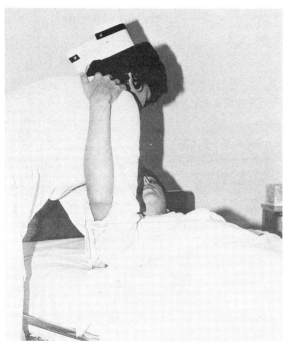

Fig. 33-1 Encourage the patient to push with both feet if possible.

Using another nurse to assist makes the procedure smoother for the patient. Also, the nurse reduces the risk of injury.

VOCABULARY

- Define the following words:

cradle   slumped

SUGGESTED ACTIVITIES

- Working in student nurse groups, practice moving another student up in bed. Students should evaluate each other's skill in practicing good posture and good body mechanics.

- Find out what self-help devices are used routinely on the orthopedic service of the hospital. How do they operate? Under what conditions are they usually ordered?

REVIEW

Select the *best* answer.

1. A nurse who is planning to move a weak or heavy patient up in bed should
    a. raise the foot of the bed
    b. raise the head of the bed
    c. place a pillow under the patient's knees
    d. ask another nurse for assistance

2. The patient can help with moving up in bed by
    a. flexing the knees and pushing with the feet
    b. holding on to the sides of the bed
    c. leaning back on the elbows
    d. holding the pillow under the head

3. The nurse should stand with the feet apart in order to
    a. keep the bed from sliding
    b. establish a broader base of support
    c. better use the back muscles
    d. shift the weight from the front to the back leg

4. To move a patient up in bed, the nurse places her hands under the patient's
    a. knees and neck   c. back and shoulders
    b. hips and neck   d. head and knees

5. Moving the patient up in bed is easier when the
    a. patient decides when to begin
    b. patient and nurse move together on a given signal
    c. nurse shifts from the front leg to the back
    d. nurse keeps the knees locked

unit 34 assisting the patient to a sitting position

OBJECTIVES

After studying this unit, the student will be able to:

- Describe the purpose of dangling.

- Explain at least one use of good body mechanics while assisting the patient to sit up in bed.

- Explain three safety precautions used in assisting the patient to dangle.

Changing from the horizontal recumbent position to a sitting position affects the patient's circulation. At times, this change will make the patient dizzy. The nurse should stay with a patient even though the patient feels well. Sitting unattended or unprotected may result in a fall.

SITTING UP IN BED

The patient may have to sit up in bed for a physical examination, to eat or just to rest in a different position. This position may be difficult to maintain for a weak or elderly patient. The nurse should elevate the head of the bed and support the patient with pillows. The nurse should also stay at the bedside unless the patient seems able to sit alone.

PROCEDURE

1. Greet the patient and explain the procedure.

2. Raise the siderail on the opposite side of the bed.

   If the patient is sitting up to eat or read, move the patient up in bed and raise the head of the bed as much as possible. For a physical exam do not elevate the bed.

3. Stand at the side of the bed and face the head of the bed.

4. Place your outer leg ahead of the leg nearest the bed.

   Avoid facing the patient directly to reduce the risk of infection.

5. Slide your right hand under the patient's right arm at the shoulder. Firmly grasp the back of the patient's upper arm. Slide your left arm underneath the patient's shoulders.

6. Ask the patient to hold the back of your right upper arm.

7. Standing with the knees bent, bring the patient to a sitting position.

8. Support the patient since the change of position may make the patient dizzy.

9. If the bed has been raised to allow the patient to eat, support the patient with pillows and raise the bedrail.

   A weak patient may slump easily or fall to the side.

SITTING UP TO DANGLE

Dangling is the position a patient assumes with the nurse's help in which he sits on the side of the bed with his legs hanging over the side. The physician usually orders this position when a patient is preparing to get out of bed for the first time. Under certain conditions the doctor may order the procedure each time the patient gets out of bed.

A sudden change to the upright position causes a diminished blood supply to reach the brain. Most patients who have been on bedrest must prepare to ambulate gradually. The nurse should watch for signs of fatigue, rapid pulse and pallor.

PROCEDURE

1. Assemble the needed articles:

   Bathrobe
   Bath blanket
   Footstool or chair
   Pillow
   Slippers

2. Explain the procedure to the patient.

3. Check the patient's pulse and any other vital signs the doctor may request.

   The patient's condition may not permit even mild exercise such as dangling.

4. Screen the unit.

   Provide privacy for the patient.

5. Help the patient to put on a bathrobe.

6. Bring both the patient's legs to the side of the bed. Bend the knees and allow the lower legs to hang off the bed.

7. Use both arms to bring the patient to a sitting position using the method already explained.

8. Turn and raise the patient at the same time.

   This motion should be natural since the feet are already off the bed.

9. Roll the pillow and place it firmly against the patient's back for support.

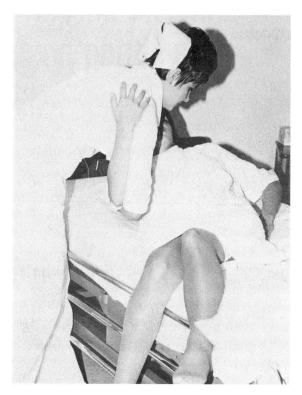

Fig. 34-1 Both of the patient's legs should hang off the bed before the head and shoulders are raised.

10. Stand next to the patient. Do not leave the patient's side.

    The patient may become dizzy at any time.

11. Instruct the patient to swing both legs gently back and forth.

12. Do not tire the patient. If desired, a chair or footstool may be placed to support the feet for a few minutes.

13. Have the patient dangle as long as is ordered by the doctor.

    Place a bath blanket around the patient's shoulders for warmth, if needed.

14. Observe the patient for dizziness or faintness. If either occurs, assist the patient back into a recumbent position. Report the patient's condition to the charge nurse.

15. When the patient becomes tired or has dangled as long as ordered, assist the patient back into bed.

16. Remove the bathrobe and slippers.

17. Place one arm around the patient's shoulders and the other under the knees. Swing the patient into bed gently.

18. If permitted, lower the head of the bed and arrange pillows and bedcovers.

19. Move the patient up in bed and place the patient in a comfortable position.

    Leave the call signal within reach of the patient.

20. Record the pulse and other vital signs taken, the time and duration the patient has dangled, and the observations of the patient's response to the procedure.

21. Report any marked change in the patient's condition to the charge nurse.

VOCABULARY

- Define the following words:

ambulate	diminished	faintness
circulation	duration	pallor
dangling		

SUGGESTED ACTIVITIES

- Working in groups, practice the sitting and dangling procedures. The students should evaluate each other's skill in practicing good posture and good body mechanics.

- Discuss which patients are likely to need to dangle before ambulating. Consider the reasons for admission and the size and age of the patients.

REVIEW

Briefly answer the following questions.

1. Why is dangling ordered before a patient is allowed to get out of bed for the first time?

2. When and why does the nurse check the patient's pulse and other vital signs before the dangling procedure?

3. What two actions should the nurse take if the patient suddenly becomes dizzy while dangling?

4. Describe the proper leg position of a nurse who is helping a patient sit up in bed.

5. Why should the nurse avoid facing the patient closely when assisting him?

unit 35 assisting the patient into the wheelchair

OBJECTIVES

After studying this unit, the student will be able to:

- Explain the procedure used to assist the patient from the bed to the wheelchair.
- Explain the purpose of assisting the patient to rest in a chair.
- Explain the ways to adjust the wheelchair.
- Describe the safety precautions used while assisting the patient into a chair.

Patients often require assistance getting up from the bed into a chair or wheelchair. The doctor may request the patient to sit in a chair to lessen the hazards of prolonged bedrest. Patients may enjoy the change of position or may find it tiring. The nurse should be sensitive to the patient's response to the procedure. At times patients need encouragement to get out of bed. The nurse's skill will lessen the patient's anxiety and make the procedure easier.

A patient may be transferred to a wheelchair instead of a chair. The wheelchair provides a change of position but also allows the patient to move around at will. The wheelchair is used primarily to transport patients. The nurse should be able to transfer a patient to a wheelchair smoothly. Using proper body mechanics lessens the strain on the patient and the nurse. If more than one nurse is required to assist the patient, it is important that the two nurses coordinate their steps. This will prevent jarring the patient.

The length of time a patient remains out of bed depends on the doctor's order. The period also depends on the number of times the patient has been out of bed and how well the activity is tolerated. The patient must be observed carefully for signs of fatigue. If the patient shows an increase in pulse rate, complains of weakness or faintness, becomes pale or shows signs of stress, the patient should be returned to bed.

PROCEDURE

1. Assemble equipment:

   Bathrobe
   2 bath blankets
   Wheelchair
   Footstool
   Pillow
   Slippers

2. Greet patient and explain procedure.

3. Screen the unit.

4. Cover the wheelchair with a bath blanket. Raise both foot pedals before placing the patient in the wheelchair.

5. Place wheelchair near bed and lock the wheels of the chair.

   A third person is needed to hold the chair if it has no locks.

6. Lock the wheels of the bed.

7. Fanfold the top bedcovers to the foot of the bed.

Drape the patient with a bath blanket to prevent exposure.

8. Elevate the head of the bed.

9. Dress the patient in a bathrobe and slippers.

10. Place a footstool at the side of the bed.

11. Assist the patient to sit up and dangle.

    Give the patient time to rest at the side of the bed before the transfer to the wheelchair.

12. Face the patient and steady the footstool with one foot. Have the patient place both feet on the center of the stool. Place his hands on your shoulders.

13. Place your hands on the rib cage of the patient under the arms. Raise the patient slightly so that he can slide off the edge of the bed and stand on the stool.

    Encourage the patient to use your shoulders for support.

14. While keeping hands in same position, help the patient step to the floor. Turn the patient slowly until his back is toward the wheelchair.

15. Place one foot in front of the other, bend the knees and lower patient gradually to a sitting position in the wheelchair. Arrange the robe smoothly.

    Lower the patient completely before releasing your hold. The patient can use the arms of the wheelchair for support.

16. Cover the patient with a bath blanket. Lower the foot pedals and place the patient's feet on them.

    Be sure the patient's feet do not fall under the pedals. The feet may be injured if they hang down while the chair is in motion.

17. Check the patient's pulse and observe for signs of pain, weakness or faintness.

    If the patient is unable to continue, request assistance to return the patient to bed.

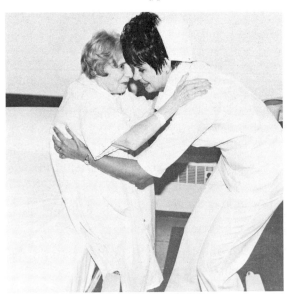

(A) The patient can grasp the nurse's shoulders for support.

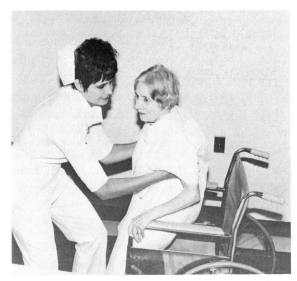

(B) Placing both hands on the wheelchair helps the patient position herself in the seat.

Fig. 35-1 Assisting the patient into a wheelchair

18. Support the patient with pillows and fasten the patient in the chair with a seat belt.

    NOTE: Never transport patients or leave them unattended without taking these measures.

19. If the patient is sitting up for a rest and is not able to move the chair, reposition the chair and lock the wheels.

    Failure to take safety precautions may result in legal problems for the nurse should the patient be injured.

20. Teach patients who are able, to unlock the wheels and move the wheelchair around the room.

    Leave the signal cord, drinking water, and other desired articles within reach of the patient.

21. If the patient is sitting in the room, check the patient's position and condition frequently. Assist the patient back to bed when the patient tires or sits for the prescribed time.

22. Record the time and duration of a patient's sitting period. For patients resting or being transported in the wheelchair, record the patient's response to the change in position. Record the pulse rate and any unusual observations.

    Report unusual observations to the nurse. Report conditions which could lead to a fall.

VOCABULARY

- Define the following words:

    legal   sensitive   stress

SUGGESTED ACTIVITY

- Working in groups with other students practice helping the patient from bed to wheelchair and from wheelchair to bed.

REVIEW

Briefly answer the following questions.

1. Why is it beneficial for patients to get out of bed into a chair?

2. What three things determine how long the patient should remain in the chair?

3. For the patient, what advantage does the wheelchair have over a regular chair?

4. Name three steps in preparing the wheelchair, prior to transferring the patient into it.

5. In what position should the foot pedals remain while the patient is being lowered into the wheelchair?

6. Where does the patient place the hands when moving to a standing position on the footstool?

7. What problems result for the nurse if the lack of safety precautions causes a patient injury?

8. Name three safety precautions to use for a weak patient resting in a wheelchair.

9. What function does the footstool perform?

10. Name two ways a patient may feel about preparing to sit up in a chair.

unit 36 moving the patient from the bed to a stretcher

OBJECTIVES

After studying this unit, the student will be able to:

- Identify the steps used to transfer a patient from a bed to a stretcher.

- Identify the use of good body mechanics while performing the transfer.

- Identify ways to reduce the patient's fear of this transfer.

Transferring the patient from the bed to the stretcher is a common hospital procedure. It is used to transport patients to the X-ray department, to the operating room or to other patient units in the hospital. At times the patient rests on the stretcher while the mattress of the bed is being cleaned or turned. Hospitals and other health facilities often use stretchers with emergency care. The nurse should become smooth and efficient in transferring the patient. An injured or seriously ill patient cannot tolerate the extra time and effort spent on a poor transfer.

Care must be taken to avoid jarring or injuring the patient. Use of good body mechanics prevents strain on the nurse and the patient. If the patient is helpless or unconscious, more people are needed to make the transfer. Many patients feel insecure during this procedure. It is essential that the patient be handled gently and skillfully in order to dispel any fears the patient may have. Using signals and explaining the steps to the patient helps reduce anxiety.

PROCEDURE

1. Prepare stretcher according to hospital policy and take it to the unit.

2. Greet patient and explain procedure.

    Be sure to check the patient's ID bracelet.

3. Screen the unit.

4. Cover patient with bath blanket. Fanfold top bedclothes to foot of bed.

    Avoid unnecessary exposure.

5. Place the stretcher next to the bed. Elevate the bed to the height of the stretcher.

6. Lock the wheels of both the bed and the stretcher.

    Be sure the head of the bed and stretcher line up. No space should exist between the two surfaces.

7. Request the help of two other team members. One should stand at the head of the bed. At least one nursing team member should be on one side of the bed and the other should be standing at the side of the stretcher.

8. Loosen the drawsheet from under the mattress and roll the edges in towards the patient from both sides.

    Roll the drawsheet close to the patient and lean over the bed so the drawsheet can be held close to the body.

9. Ask the person at the head of the bed to support the patient's head. This is done by lifting slightly when the transfer takes place.

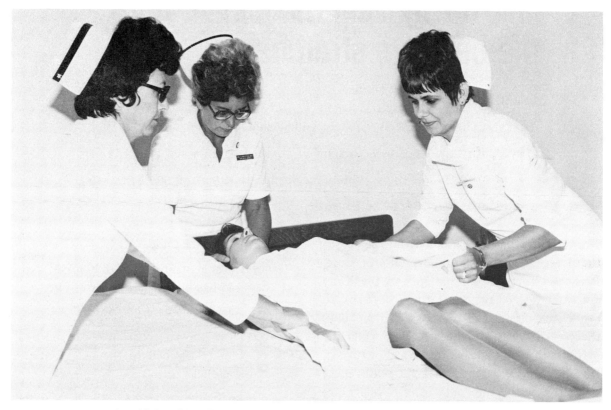

Fig. 36-1 Lifting the patient onto a stretcher requires at least three people.

A weak patient's head may drop when the rest of the body is lifted. If needed, a fourth person can lift the feet.

10. Have the two persons on the sides hold the rolled drawsheet. On a given signal, all lift to transfer the patient onto the stretcher.

Lift high enough to clear the bump between the bed and stretcher.

11. Place a pillow under the patient's head and raise the siderails of the stretcher.

Do not allow the patient's arms to hang off the sides.

12. If the patient is being transported, use one person at the end and foot of the stretcher.

Transport patients slowly around corners. To go down inclines, walk backwards holding the lower end of the stretcher.

13. Record the time, the destination of the patient and any observations made during the transfer.

To transfer the patient from the stretcher back to the bed, use the same procedure. If the bedding on the stretcher has changed, use the sheet on it to lift the patient. Another drawsheet can be rolled under the patient if needed. The patient may be tired and less tolerant with the transfer back to bed. Be gentle and work slowly.

VOCABULARY

- Define the following words:

    insecurity   unconscious

SUGGESTED ACTIVITIES

- With a group of student nurses, practice the stretcher transfer. Assemble three assistants and one person to role play as a patient. Assume the patient cannot help with the transfer. Practice until the transfer is smooth and efficient.

- Using a drawsheet, practice moving a person who is in bed. Note that the farther away from the patient the drawsheet is held, the greater the pull on your back muscles. Practice good mechanics.

REVIEW

Select the *best* answer.

1. One safety measure in a bed to stretcher transfer is

   a. locking the wheels of both the stretcher and bed
   b. leaving at least one inch between the two surfaces to absorb bumps
   c. standing on the side near the head of the bed
   d. standing on the side near the foot of the bed

2. The stretcher is positioned next to the bed so that the

   a. heads are at right angles to each other
   b. stretcher is slightly lower than the bed
   c. heads line up with each other
   d. siderails lock

3. To lift the patient the nurses should hold the rolled drawsheet

   a. near the edges of the bed
   b. as close to the patient as possible
   c. at a right angle to the bed
   d. with the hands spread far apart

4. One method of reducing strain on the nurse is to

   a. keep the knees straight
   b. only lift light patients
   c. kneel on the patient's bed
   d. lean over and hold the drawsheet close to nurse's own body

5. The nurse can help reduce the patient's fear of the stretcher transfer by

   a. using a smooth and efficient technique
   b. explaining the steps to the patient
   c. asking other team members to be gentle
   d. all of the above

SELF-EVALUATION VI

A. Select the *best* answer.

1. A patient can be spared the sense of helplessness if the

    a. nurse introduces the patient to others
    b. patient has a special nurse
    c. patient has visitors constantly
    d. patient is permitted to do as much as he is able

2. Prolonged bedrest may be complicated by

    a. loss of muscle tone
    b. contracture of muscles
    c. decubiti
    d. all of the above

3. The patient can gradually adjust to an upright position by

    a. sitting with the head between the knees
    b. dangling before standing up
    c. resting in Trendelenburg position
    d. resting in Sims' position

4. When moving a patient the most important thing to be considered is

    a. the safety of the patient and the nurse
    b. the appearance of the patient
    c. economy of time
    d. position of the bedcovers

5. The best means of maintaining good muscle tone in a patient is to

    a. encourage the patient to help in transfers and exercise if permitted
    b. give alcohol rub frequently
    c. give hot soaks
    d. give muscle relaxants

6. If the patient finds one position most comfortable the patient should

    a. remain in that position
    b. no matter how comfortable, move or be assisted to move at least every hour
    c. make certain the posture is good for a few hours
    d. sleep in that position

7. The length of time a patient remains out of bed will depend upon

    a. physician's order
    b. the patient's tolerance
    c. how many times he has been out of bed
    d. all of the above

8. The patient needs to be returned to bed sooner than planned if

    a. visitors arrive
    b. there is a small change in the pulse rate
    c. the patient complains of weakness or faintness
    d. the patient wants to read in bed

9. The patient's muscles receive more stimulation

    a. if the nurse moves the body into position
    b. if the patient moves without help from the nurse
    c. from sitting up in bed rather than dangling
    d. if the patient enjoys the activity

10. A chair or footstool is placed at the side of the bed when the patient dangles

    a. to prevent the patient from falling asleep
    b. to provide a resting place for the patient's feet
    c. to keep personal articles within reach
    d. for the patient to sit on if desired

B. Complete the following statements.

1. The footboard is used to prevent _____.

2. The device used to eliminate the weight of bedcovers on a certain area of the body is called a _____.

3. The least number of people needed to lift a weak patient from the bed to the stretcher is _____.

4. When moving a patient up in bed, the head of the bed should be in a position which is _____.

5. The purpose of dangling is to _____.

SECTION VII THE PATIENT'S PERSONAL HYGIENE

unit 37 offering the bedpan or urinal

OBJECTIVES

After studying this unit, the student will be able to:

- Identify the principles to follow in giving and removing the bedpan.
- Give 3 reasons why a patient may not be able to use the bedpan or urinal.

Eliminating wastes is usually the patient's first activity in the morning. Patients who are not able to get up to use the bathroom, require a bedpan or urinal. Activities included in morning care usually occur in the following order:

- Offering the bedpan or urinal
- Washing the patient's face and hands
- Giving oral hygiene
- Serving breakfast
- Giving the bed bath
- Giving a back rub
- Combing the hair
- Dressing the patient

The routine planned for morning care is similar to the routine followed by most persons who are able to care for themselves. The nurse, however, should not assume the patient needs to eliminate wastes at an accepted time. Some persons do not have bowel movements every morning; others may not have the necessity or habit of voiding frequently. Hospital routines help organize the activities of patients and hospital staff. However, they should remain as flexible as possible.

The elimination of waste material is a necessary and natural process of the body. However, patients often do not adjust easily to using a bedpan or urinal. To promote satisfactory elimination, the nurse should provide privacy for the patient. The patient should be placed on the bedpan as comfortably as possible and left alone with the signal cord within reach. If the patient cannot be left alone, the nurse should be considerate and not attract attention. Besides the awkward position and shyness, other conditions may affect the patient's ability to void. A decrease in physical activity, changes in diet, and certain medications may cause urinary problems, constipation, or diarrhea. The attitude of the nurse can help the patient cope with these problems.

OFFERING THE BEDPAN

Nurses should always provide the bedpan promptly after being asked for it. Patients should also be offered its use before treatments. A male nurse or attendant usually cares for the personal needs of the male patient. Since a male is not always available, the female nurse should learn to perform this procedure with tact. When the use of the bedpan causes fatigue, it should be reported to the physician. In many cases, the use of a bedside commode may cause less strain.

PROCEDURE

1. Assemble equipment as it is used:

   Bedpan and cover
   Toilet tissue
   Basin of warm water
   Soap
   Washcloth
   Towel

2. Greet patient and explain procedure.

3. Screen the unit.

4. Place the bedpan on the bedside chair. Put tissue on the bedside stand within easy reach of the patient.

   Put bedpan on foot of bed if there is no chair.

5. Warm the bedpan by running hot water into it and emptying it. A cold bedpan may discourage voiding or defecation. In hot weather, talcum powder may be used on the bedpan to prevent the patient from sticking to it.

6. Fold top bedcovers back at a right angle without exposing the patient.

   Pad bedpan with folded towel if patient is thin or has a pressure sore.

7. Assist the patient to lift the gown while keeping top covers in place.

8. Ask patient to flex the knees and raise the buttocks by putting weight on the heels. If needed, put one hand under the small of the patient's back and lift gently. Place bedpan under the hips with the other hand.

   If patient is unable to raise buttocks, two nurses may be needed to lift patient. The pan may be inserted by rolling patient to one side, placing the bedpan and rolling patient back on it. The pan must be held in place with one hand as patient rolls back on it.

Patient's buttocks should rest on rounded shelf of bedpan. The narrow end should face the foot of the bed.

9. Raise head of bed to comfortable height.

   Unless condition indicates otherwise.

10. Make sure signal cord is within easy reach of patient.

    Leave patient alone unless the condition does not permit it.

11. Fill basin with warm water. Obtain soap, washcloth and towel. Wait until the patient signals for assistance.

    Answer patient's signal immediately.

12. Ask patient to flex knees and rest weight on heels. Place one hand under small of patient's back and lift gently to help patient raise buttocks off bedpan. Take bedpan with other hand. Cover bedpan and place on chair.

    If patient is unable to raise buttocks, two nurses may be needed to assist the patient.

13. Clean buttocks and rectal area as necessary. Discard tissue in bedpan unless specimen is to be collected. Cover bedpan.

14. Encourage patient to wash the hands and freshen up after the procedure.

    Change drawsheet and the patient's gown if necessary.

15. Take bedpan to bathroom or utility room.

    Observe contents. Measure and record the output if ordered.

16. Empty bedpan. Rinse with cold water. Clean with warm soapy water. If available, use a mechanical hopper.

Cold water prevents protein from coagulating and sticking to bedpan.

17. Rinse, dry, and cover bedpan. Place inside patient's bedside table.

Use bedpan sterilizer or send to central supply if ordered by hospital policy.

18. Chart the amount and character of any solid waste or urine voided Record any unusual observations.

Report any unusual observations immediately to the supervising nurse.

OFFERING THE URINAL

A patient who requires a urinal can in many cases use it without assistance. Many patients only require the nurse's help to empty the urinal. The nurse should offer to help before assuming the patient can handle the procedure alone. A respectful manner is needed to make the patient comfortable. Use the basic steps explained for offering a bedpan.

VOCABULARY

- Define the following words:

    commode   constipation   diarrhea

SUGGESTED ACTIVITY

- Obtain the assistance of another student. Have this student role play a helpless patient lying in bed. Use the procedure described to assist the patient onto the bedpan.

REVIEW

A. Select the *best* answer.

1. The activity which usually begins the patient's morning care is

    a. eating breakfast
    b. taking a shower
    c. taking medications
    d. eliminating wastes

2. A weak patient may be able to void without help if he uses a

    a. basin
    b. urinal
    c. bedside commode
    d. bathroom toilet

3. The bedpan is rinsed with cold water after use to

    a. prevent wastes from sticking to the pan
    b. kill microorganisms quickly
    c. make the pan easier to handle
    d. help the soap adhere better

4. When the nurse positions a patient on a bedpan, the patient can help by

    a. folding the bedcovers to the end of the bed
    b. leaning back on the elbows
    c. putting weight on the heels and raising the buttocks
    d. exposing the buttocks

5. The nurse can show consideration for the patient's privacy by

    a. putting a Do Not Disturb sign outside the door

    b. keeping an extra blanket in the room

    c. not exposing the patient during the procedure

    d. talking courteously with the patient's family

B.   Briefly answer the following questions.

1. Name two reasons the patient may have difficulty in using a bedpan or urinal.

2. What would you do if the patient refused the bedpan before morning care?

unit 38 oral hygiene

OBJECTIVES

After studying this unit, the student will be able to:

- List the benefits of oral hygiene.

- Explain the care of dentures.

- Describe the steps used to give a helpless patient oral hygiene.

Oral hygiene or care of the mouth and teeth ideally should be performed at least three times a day, depending on the needs of the patient. Keeping the mouth as clean as possible helps to maintain the mouth, teeth, and gums in healthy condition. Oral hygiene aids in preventing caries and disease, stimulates the appetite, and increases the patient's sense of well-being.

ROUTINE ORAL HYGIENE

Giving the patient oral hygiene is an important part of routine morning care. Some patients prefer to brush their teeth or rinse their mouth both before and after breakfast. The nurse should help patients keep their own routines as much as possible. Providing a patient with the items needed is often the most help a patient needs. Encourage patients to care for themselves to the extent that they are able.

PROCEDURE

1. Assemble equipment:

   Toothbrush
   Toothpaste or tooth powder
   Mouthwash solution in cup
   Emesis basin
   Paper bag
   Bath towel
   Drinking tube
   Tissues
   Cup of fresh water

2. Greet patient and explain procedure.

3. Screen the unit.

4. Raise back of bed so that patient can sit up for procedure.

   Check the doctor's order to see that raising the head of the bed has not been prohibited.

5. Place bath towel over patient's gown and bedcovers.

6. Pour water over toothbrush and put toothpaste on brush. Give brush to patient.

   If the patient is not able, the nurse should brush the patient's teeth carefully and thoroughly.

7. Give patient rinse water in a cup.

   Have patient use emesis basin to expel the rinse water. Help raise the head if the patient is in supine position. Hold the emesis basin under patient's chin for return of the fluid. If patient finds this procedure difficult in the supine position, turn the patient's head to one side with emesis basin near the chin.

8. Offer mouthwash once the mouth is rinsed well.

9. Remove basin. Give the patient a tissue to wipe the mouth and chin. Discard the tissue in a paper bag.

Assist the patient if necessary.

10. Remove the towel.

11. Rinse the toothbrush with water.

12. Clean and replace equipment according to hospital policy.

13. Record: Time
    Procedure: Oral Hygiene
    Observations

Note condition of gums, tongue, teeth and lips. Report unusual observations immediately to supervising nurse.

In many hospitals routine procedures are not recorded unless there is an unusual condition noted. In others, morning and evening routines are recorded in detail.

CARE OF DENTURES

When a patient wears dentures, the nurse is responsible to see that they are not lost or broken. Extreme care must be used when handling dentures. When the patient is not wearing them, dentures should be kept in the bedside table in a container labeled with the patient's name. Vulcanite dentures should be covered with a mild antiseptic solution. Plastic dentures should be kept dry.

Dentures are cleaned in much the same way as natural teeth, with a toothbrush and tooth powder or toothpaste. The container for the dentures should also be cleaned and labeled clearly. The patient may feel embarrassed about wearing dentures. Therefore, the nurse should provide privacy when they are removed and cleaned.

PROCEDURE

1. Assemble equipment:

    Tissues
    Emesis basin
    Toothbrush or denture brush
    Toothpaste or tooth powder
    Gauze squares
    Denture cup

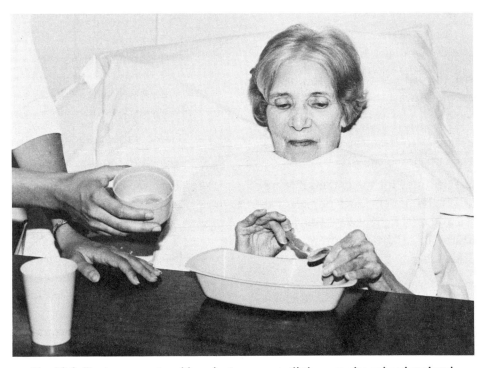

Fig. 38-1 Dentures are stored in a denture cup until they are cleaned and replaced.

2. Greet patient and explain procedure.

3. Screen the unit.

   Provide privacy. The patient may not want to remove the dentures in the presence of the nurse. Allow the patient to clean dentures privately if requested.

4. Ask patient to remove dentures. Give tissue to patient.

   If patient cannot remove the dentures easily, the nurse should do it slowly and carefully.

5. Place dentures in denture cup padded with gauze squares. Take them to the bathroom or utility room.

6. Put toothpaste or tooth powder on toothbrush. Place dentures in palm of hand and hold them under a gentle stream of warm water. Brush until all surfaces are clean.

7. Rinse dentures thoroughly under cold running water.

8. Place dentures in clean denture cup and take them back to the bedside.

9. Assist the patient to rinse the mouth with mouthwash before dentures are replaced.

10. Use a tissue to hand the dentures back to the patient.

    Insert dentures for the patient if necessary. If the patient does not want to replace them right away, place the dentures in a labeled denture cup in bedside table.

11. Clean and replace equipment according to hospital policy.

12. Record: Time
    Procedure: Denture Care
    Observations

Report any mouth or gum irritations caused by the dentures to the supervising nurse.

ORAL HYGIENE FOR THE HELPLESS PATIENT

Special oral hygiene is needed for cleaning the mouth of the helpless patient. This procedure should be performed at least three times a day. If the patient is unconscious, has a high temperature or facial paralysis, lemon-glycerin swabs are used to swab the tongue, lips and mucous membranes of the mouth. This prevents the mouth and lips from becoming dry. It also helps prevent sordes. *Sordes* are foul, brown secretions which form into crusts around the lips and teeth.

PROCEDURE

1. Assemble equipment on a tray:

   Cotton applicators
   4 tongue blades
   4 gauze squares
   Tissues
   Mouth solution as ordered
   Face towel
   Lemon-glycerin swabs (or petroleum jelly if swabs are not available)
   Emesis basin
   Drinking tube

2. Greet patient and explain procedure.

3. Screen the unit.

4. Turn the patient to the side.

5. Put a towel under the patient's chin.
   Use a protective pad if needed.

6. Pad tongue blade with gauze. Open gauze square and fold into a triangle. Place the end of the tongue blade at the apex of the triangle and roll firmly. Fold excess gauze neatly over top of tongue blade. Wrap in bandage and tie the ends.

7. Moisten padded blade with mouth-wash and thoroughly swab the teeth, tongue, roof and sides of the mouth.

   It may be necessary to hold the patient's mouth open by using another padded tongue blade.

8. Help patient to rinse mouth with mouthwash and then with fresh water. Dry area around the mouth with towel.

9. Remove gauze and rewrap tongue blade.

   Discard gauze in basin.

10. Apply the lemon-glycerin swab to the tongue, lips and mucous membrane of the mouth. Remove excess solution around mouth with tissue.

    If petroleum jelly is applied, use it sparingly and remove excess with a tissue.

11. Remove the protective towel.

12. Clean and replace equipment according to hospital policy.

13. Record: Time
    Procedure: Oral Hygiene
    Observations

    Report any unusual observations to the supervising nurse.

VOCABULARY

- Define the following words:

apex	dentures	paralysis
appetite	glycerin	sordes
caries	oral	vulcanite

SUGGESTED ACTIVITIES

- If possible, obtain a pair of dentures or partials. Practice brushing them and clean all the surfaces completely.

- Discuss with the instructor the value of using disclosing tablets. These tablets are chewed after brushing to color food particles or areas missed during brushing. A second brushing can remove the coloring and the remaining particles or film. Is the use of these tablets practical for hospital care?

REVIEW

Briefly answer the following questions.

1. Name three benefits of oral hygiene.

2. What kind of container is used for the storage of dentures when they are not in use?

3. Why are lemon-glycerin swabs applied to the inside of the mouth and lips of an unconscious patient?

4. How does the nurse position the helpless patient when giving oral hygiene?

5. What simple piece of equipment is used to clean the mouth membranes with mouthwash. How is it prepared for this use?

unit 39 the bed bath

OBJECTIVES

After studying this unit, the student will be able to:

- Identify the benefits a bed bath provides for the patient.
- Explain the procedure for giving a complete bed bath.
- List in proper order the areas to be washed when giving a bed bath.

A bed bath is a complete bath the patient receives while lying in bed. Patients who are weak, seriously ill or have certain heart conditions may not be able to bathe in the shower or tub. The nurse must learn to give a bed bath without tiring the patient. If done correctly a bath refreshes the patient greatly. Baths also stimulate circulation in the skin and the tissues underneath, and remove perspiration and body discharges.

The nurse who gives the bed bath should encourage the patient to assist if his condition permits. This provides exercise and reduces any feelings of helplessness that the patient may have. The bed bath can also provide time for conversation with the patient. The patient's ability and desire for self-help may be revealed during this time. Knowing the patient better can help the nurse detect when the patient is tired, or in need of something.

A complete daily bath is not advisable for all patients. Elderly patients have a decrease in production of perspiration and natural oils which keep the skin moist. As a result, these patients need not wash as frequently. Instead of a complete bath, the nurse may give a partial bath. In a partial bath, the face, arms, hands, and back are washed. With either the complete or the partial bed bath, rubbing the back with lotion makes the patient more comfortable.

PREPARING TO GIVE A BED BATH

Assembling the needed supplies before the bath saves time and effort later. Leaving the patient during the bed bath procedure should be avoided. Besides gathering the items needed, the bed and room must be prepared. The nurse can give better care by being organized.

PROCEDURE

1. Assemble equipment:

    Bed linen (linen pack)
    Bath blanket
    Laundry bag or hamper
    Basin of water 105-115°F (41-46°C)
    Bath thermometer
    Soap and soap dish
    Washcloth
    Face towel
    Bath towel
    Gown
    Lotion, powder

2. Greet patient and explain procedure.

3. Make sure windows and door are closed to prevent chilling the patient.

4. Screen the unit.

5. Put towels and linen pack on chair in order of use. Place laundry hamper in a place which is easy to reach.

6. Offer bedpan or urinal.

Empty and clean before proceeding with bath. Wash hands.

7. Lower back of bed if permitted.

8. Loosen top bedcovers and place a bath blanket over them. Slide the top bedclothes out from under the bath blanket.

   Avoid exposing the patient.

9. Leave one pillow under the patient's head. Place any other pillows on a chair.

10. Leaving the bath blanket in place, remove patient's gown. Place it in the laundry hamper.

    Check the gown for valuables which belong to the patient.

11. Remove dressings or bandages if permitted.

    Removal must be permitted by the doctor. Check with the supervising nurse, if in doubt.

12. Fill a basin 2/3 full with water at temperature of 105-115°F (41-46°C)

    Test water with bath thermometer.

13. Ask patient to move to the side of the bed nearest the nurse.

    Assist if necessary. Practice good body mechanics and do not expose the patient.

14. Fold a towel over upper edge of bath blanket to keep it dry.

15. Place the water and towels near the bed and see that the patient is ready to begin.

WASHING THE PATIENT

Nurses should be careful that the water is the correct temperature throughout the bath. At some point in the bath, a water change may be needed. Dripping water on the patient should also be avoided. Using cool water or exposing the patient may cause chills and make the bath unpleasant.

PROCEDURE

1. Wet the washcloth. Squeeze out the excess water.

2. Form a mitt by folding the washcloth around one hand.

   The washcloth mitt prevents ends from dragging across the patient and prevents water from dripping on the patient and bed.

3. Wash each eye carefully. Start from the inner corner and brush outward.

   Always wash the eyes first since the cleanest water is needed for them.

4. Wash and rinse patient's face, ears and neck. Use face towel to dry.

   Allow patient to wash face and hands if condition permits.

   Make sure all soap is removed, since soap film may cause skin irritation.

5. Expose only one of the patient's arms at a time. Protect bed with bath towel or protective pad placed underneath the arm. Wash, rinse and dry arm and hand. Repeat for other arm.

   Be sure axillae are clean and dry. Apply deodorant at this time or when bath has been completed.

6. Put bath towel over patient's chest. Then fold bath blanket to waist. Under the towel, wash, rinse and dry chest.

   Observe female patient's breasts without exposing them. Note any irritation or lumps. Rinse and dry folds under breasts carefully to avoid irritating the skin.

7. To cover patient's chest and abdomen, place a bath towel lengthwise under the bath blanket. Then fold the bath blanket down to the patient's waist. Wash, rinse and dry abdomen under towel. Fold bath blanket up to cover abdomen and chest. Slide towel out from beneath bath blanket.

Make sure creases and folds of skin are clean and dry.

8. Ask patient to flex one knee. Fold bath blanket up to expose thigh, leg and foot. Protect bed with bath towel. Put bath basin on towel and place the patient's foot in the basin. Wash and rinse the leg and foot.

When moving leg, support it properly, grasping heel of foot with one hand.

Note any color changes or irritated areas on toes and heels.

9. Move the basin to the other side of the bed and wash the other leg in the same manner.

10. Take basin from the bed before drying the leg and foot.

11. Change water and check for correct temperature with bath thermometer.

Change water as often as needed. It may be necessary to change water before this point in the patient's bath.

12. Help patient to turn on the side, facing away from the nurse. Place a bath towel lengthwise on the bed next to the patient's back. Wash, rinse and dry neck, back and buttocks.

The patient may lie on the abdomen if he wishes.

Use long, firm strokes when washing the back. Examine the body areas for redness or skin breakdown.

13. Give back rub now or at a later time.

If the patient is tiring from the bath, the back rub can be given later.

14. Help patient return to the back-lying position. Ask if the patient is able to complete the bath by washing the genitalia.

Most patients prefer to complete this part of the bath themselves.

15. If the patient is able, place the washcloth, soap, basin and towel within reach.

Provide privacy.

16. If the patient is unconscious or clearly unable, complete the bath without the patient's assistance.

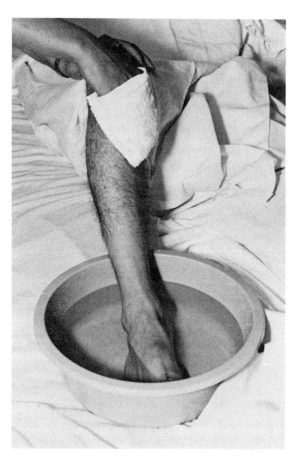

Fig. 39-1 If the patient is able, he may soak his foot while the leg is being washed.

Nurses taking care of patients of the opposite sex should display an attitude which can put the patient at ease.

17. Assist the patient into a clean gown.

18. Apply lotion to dry skin areas.

Diabetic patients should have lotion applied between the toes and on rough areas to prevent the skin from cracking.

19. Assist the patient to apply cosmetics, if desired.

20. Care for the patient's nails, if needed.

File nails straight across. Do not round edges and do not break the skin. Do not push back cuticle because it is easily injured and infected.

21. Continue with other morning care activities before changing the patient's bed linen.

Shaving, care of the hair, and giving a back rub may be needed before linen is changed.

22. Clean and replace equipment.

23. Report and record any change in the patient's skin condition.

VOCABULARY

- Define the following words:

    cuticle   genitalia   partial

SUGGESTED ACTIVITIES

- Discuss with the instructor the extra nursing skills which should be used while giving a bed bath. Consider the following topics.

    - Beginning decubiti

    - Range of motion exercises

    - Directed conversation

- Practice the procedure for giving foot care to a diabetic patient. Ask another student to role play as the patient. Wash and dry the feet carefully. Give cuticle and nail care as described in the procedure. Discuss why diabetics need special nail and skin care.

REVIEW

Select the *best* answer.

1. A complete daily bath is not advised for patients who are

    a. irritable
    b. children under two years
    c. elderly
    d. helpless

2. The purpose of giving a bed bath is to

    a. refresh the patient
    b. stimulate the circulation in the skin
    c. remove perspiration and body discharges
    d. all of the above

3. Patients who should not have a complete bath should instead

    a. take a shower
    b. have a partial bath
    c. use the tub
    d. take a sitz bath

4. The patient, if able, should assist with the bed bath to

    a. make it easier for the nurse
    b. obtain mild exercise
    c. assure getting a better bath
    d. reduce the time spent in the hospital

5. When giving foot care, the toenails should be cut

    a. straight across
    b. round at the nail edges
    c. only with bandage scissors
    d. only with nail clippers

6. When washing the patient's back, the nurse should use

    a. short, pressured strokes
    b. the heel of the hand
    c. a light, wisping motion
    d. long, firm strokes

7. When giving special skin care to the diabetic patient, remember to

    a. gently rub lotion between the toes
    b. give the patient two partial baths a day
    c. scrub dry areas extra well with soap and water
    d. help the patient stay in one comfortable position

8. The two pieces of linen which are used to prevent unnecessary exposure during a bed bath are the

    a. top sheet and spread
    b. bath blanket and towel
    c. towel and top sheet
    d. bath blanket and top sheet

9. To prepare to give a bed bath, the nurse should

    a. place the water and towels near the bedside
    b. test the water with a bath thermometer
    c. make sure the windows are closed
    d. do all of the above

10. The nurse avoids dripping water on the patient by

    a. filling only 1/3 of the basin with water
    b. holding a towel under the washcloth at all times
    c. folding the washcloth into a mitt
    d. using only a partially wet washcloth

unit 40 the back rub

OBJECTIVES

After studying this unit, the student will be able to:

- Describe the benefits of a back rub.

- Identify basic principles about back rubs.

The back rub is usually given as part of the patient's routine morning care. It also may help relax the patient in the evening or during the day after a change of position. Most back rubs require three to five minutes to complete. The nurse should gauge the time to the patient's needs.

A back rub will stimulate circulation in the skin and thus aid in preventing decubiti. Increasing circulation over bony areas is especially important in preventing decubiti. The back rub can awaken and refresh or soothe and relax the patient. The speed and direction of the strokes used help evoke the desired result. Any back rub should include long, smooth strokes since these increase the blood supply to the skin.

PROCEDURE

1. Assemble equipment:

    Basin of water 105-115°F (41-46°C)
    Bath towel
    Washcloth
    Soap
    Body powder
    Lotion

2. Greet patient and explain procedure.

    Nurses should be sure their fingernails are short enough so as not to scratch the patient.

3. Screen the unit.

4. Arrange the patient's gown so that the back is exposed.

5. Assist the patient into a prone position.

6. Wash the patient's back with soap and warm water. Dry thoroughly.

    If the back rub follows soon after the bed bath, this washing is unnecessary.

7. Apply lotion to your own hands and rub it between the hands until it is warm.

    Applying cold lotion to the back is unpleasant for the patient.

8. Rub the lotion into the skin of the back beginning at the base of spine and moving up the center. Continue around the shoulders and down the sides of the back. Repeat the stroke four times beginning and ending at the base of the spine.

    Apply more pressure on the upstroke than on the downstroke.

9. Follow the long smooth strokes with a variation shown in figure 40-2. Use the long smooth strokes moving up the center but use a circular motion on the downstroke. Repeat four times.

    Continue from one variation to the next without stopping.

10. A second variation on the downstroke requires the nurse to make a small

circular motion with the palm of the hand. This movement seen in figure 40-3 should also be repeated four times.

Apply more lotion if needed.

11. Return to using only the long, smooth strokes both up and down the back. Continue rubbing in this manner for three to five minutes.

12. Wipe away excess lotion and apply powder to the patient's back.

If the patient's skin is dry, use of powder may not be advisable.

13. Tie the patient's gown together in the back and assist the patient into a comfortable position.

14. Report and record any red areas seen on the patient's skin.

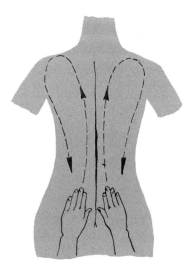

Fig. 40-1 Soothing strokes

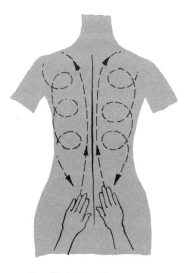

Fig. 40-2 Circular movement

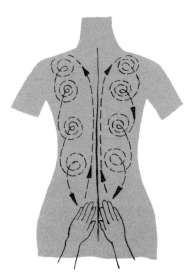

Fig. 40-3 Passive movement

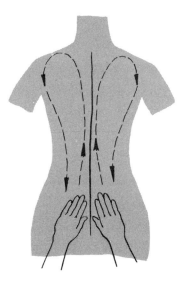

Fig. 40-4 Soothing strokes

VOCABULARY

- Define the following words:

  downstroke   passive   variation

SUGGESTED ACTIVITIES

- If a mannequin is available, demonstrate the back rub procedure.
- Discuss with the instructor other strokes which may be used in giving a back rub.

REVIEW

Briefly answer the following questions.

1. Name three times when back rubs are most commonly given.

2. What should the nurse do with the lotion before applying it to the patient's back?

3. Should more pressure be applied to the upstroke or the downstroke?

4. What condition does stimulating the circulation to bony parts help to prevent?

5. Which part of the back always receives the upward motion in the strokes described in this unit?

unit 41 the tub bath or shower

OBJECTIVES

After studying this unit, the student will be able to:

- Explain how to help the patient taking a tub bath or shower.
- Identify safety precautions to be taken.
- Give the recommended water temperatures for tub bath in Fahrenheit and Celsius degrees.

Patients who are able usually prefer a tub bath or shower to a bed bath. The doctor indicates whether the patient is allowed to use the bath facilities. Patients who use the tub or shower still require the nurse's assistance. The nurse must prepare the bathroom and gather the needed supplies. In addition, the patient should be helped to whatever extent is necessary in the judgment of the nurse.

SAFETY PRECAUTIONS

Special precautions must be taken to avoid having the patient slip in the shower or tub. CAUTION: Soap, oil, and water on the floor create a slippery surface. Patients can easily fall and injure themselves in the bathroom area. Instruct the patient to use the handrails on the walls. The patient should be shown the call signal in the bathroom and advised to use it if needed. The nurse should place a nonskid bathmat in the tub or shower.

Even though patients seem strong and alert, they should be checked at least every five minutes. Showers and baths do not need to last more than ten minutes. Patients who are taking a shower or bath after prolonged bedrest, need to be watched carefully for dizziness. These patients may also tire easily.

ASSISTING WITH A TUB BATH

The nurse should assist the patient into and out of the tub. Anyone can fall during this procedure. Weak patients should never be left unattended. The patient may become tired or dizzy, and slip causing injury. Some patients require the nurse's help throughout the bath.

PROCEDURE

1. Assemble the bath items:

   Soap
   Washcloth
   2 bath towels
   Face towel
   Bath blanket
   Bathmat
   Bath thermometer
   Bath powder
   Chair or stool
   Patient's gown, robe and slippers

2. Greet the patient and explain the procedure.

3. Take the supplies to the bathroom and prepare them for the patient.

4. Fill tub half full with water, 95-105°F (35-41°C).

   Test water temperature using a bath thermometer.

5. Assist the patient into a robe and slippers.

6. Use a wheelchair to transport the patient if the tub area is not close by.

   This conserves the patient's strength.

7. Place a nonskid bathmat in the bottom of the tub.

   Slipping in the tub is avoided.

8. Help the patient to undress and wrap in a bath blanket to prevent chilling and unnecessary exposure.

   Show the patient the call signal and explain how to use it. The safety of the patient is of primary concern.

9. Assist the patient to step into the tub.

   Give the necessary support.

10. Wash the back but encourage the patient to do the rest alone. Assist if needed, however.

    Observe the skin for areas of redness.

    If the patient shows any signs of weakness, remove the plug and let the water drain out. Allow the patient to rest and recover before assisting the patient out of the tub. Keep the patient covered with a bath towel to avoid chilling.

11. Assist the patient out of the tub. Keep the bath blanket draped around the shoulders. Dry thoroughly, powder and help the patient put on a fresh gown, robe and slippers.

12. Assist the patient back to the unit.

    Use a wheelchair if necessary.

13. Replace clean towels in the patient's unit and clean the bathtub.

14. Record the time the tub bath was taken and report any unusual observations.

ASSISTING WITH A SHOWER

A patient must show no signs of weakness before a shower is permitted. The doctor will indicate when the patient is ready for this activity. However, the nurse should also use judgment to decide whether a patient is able to shower. The patient's condition may vary throughout the day. A patient may have medical permission, however, signs of weakness, dizziness, or fatigue may require postponement of the shower. Safety precautions explained at the beginning of the unit should be reviewed. Observing safety rules in the shower helps prevent injuries.

PROCEDURE

1. Assemble supplies:

   Soap
   Washcloth
   2 bath towels
   Face towel
   Bath blanket
   Bathmat
   Bath powder
   Chair or stool
   Patient's gown, robe and slippers

2. Greet patient and explain procedure.

3. Take the supplies to the bathroom and prepare them for the patient.

4. Assist the patient into a robe and slippers. Show the patient where the shower is located.

5. Place a nonskid bathmat in the bottom of the shower.

6. Help the patient undress and wrap him in a bath blanket.

   Instruct the patient to use the call signal.

7. Assist the patient in washing if necessary.

   Observe for signs of weakness before leaving patient alone.

8. Check on the patient within five minutes.

   Do not allow the patient to remain in the shower longer than ten minutes.

9. Assist the patient to dry and dress in the gown, robe and slippers.

10. Be sure the patient is not too tired to walk back to the room. Obtain a wheelchair if signs of fatigue appear.

    Patients may tire more quickly than they realize.

11. Supply the patient's room with clean towels and bath items.

12. Record the procedure and report any unusual observations to the nurse in charge.

VOCABULARY

- Define the following words:

  nonskid   precautions   prolonged

SUGGESTED ACTIVITY

- If permitted by a doctor's order, patients on prolonged bedrest can be taken to the shower area on a special cot which rolls over the tub. Discuss with the instructor how nurses can use this equipment.

REVIEW

Select the *best* answer.

1. On a Fahrenheit thermometer, the temperature of water drawn for a tub bath registered 105°F. This is the same as

   a. 35 degrees Celsius   c. 32 degrees Celsius
   b. 41 degrees Celsius   d. 46 degrees Celsius

2. A bath blanket is necessary in order to help

   a. prevent chilling and unnecessary exposure
   b. wash large body areas and to soak sore muscles
   c. reduce itching and skin irritation
   d. prevent the patient from slipping and to make a padded seat

3. The nurse discontinues the tub bath procedure if the patient experiences

   a. exposure or chill   c. dizziness or weakness
   b. anger or fatigue   d. difficulty in walking

4. A substance which can create a slippery floor surface is

   a. soap   c. oil
   b. water   d. any of the above

5. Safety devices the patient can use in the shower area are

   a. handrails   c. nonskid bathmat
   b. call signal   d. all of the above

unit 42 daily care of the hair

OBJECTIVES

After studying this unit, the student will be able to:

- Explain how combing and brushing the hair benefits the patient's health.

- Describe the way to comb or brush properly.

- Tell why a dry shampoo may be used.

Good grooming of the hair is a part of routine morning care. Combing and brushing the hair stimulates the circulation of the scalp, helps to release the natural oils and removes loose dandruff. Brushed hair also improves the patient's appearance and usually creates a sense of well-being. Many patients are able to brush their own hair. The nurse should encourage patients who are able, to brush or comb the hair daily. Patients who seem uninterested should be assisted. A simple, friendly compliment on the patient's appearance after grooming the hair will often encourage the patient to improve grooming habits.

A dry shampoo can be used to clean the hair. It removes oils and leaves the hair soft. The style of the hair does not change. This procedure is simple and is often used instead of the regular shampoo for patients on bedrest. However, a wet shampoo may be advisable for some patients. Approval for the procedure must be obtained from the doctor. Many hospitals now have beauticians who shampoo and style hair at the bedside.

COMBING AND BRUSHING

Some patients have a very sensitive scalp; the nurse must work carefully and avoid pulling the hair. Pulling easily occurs when the hair is long and has become snarled. The nurse should not cut snarled hair. It can be unsnarled by dividing into small sections and working from the ends toward the scalp. A section of hair is held firmly with one hand, between the scalp and the comb. The other hand carefully combs out the snarls.

PROCEDURE

1. Assemble equipment:

   Towel
   Comb and brush

2. Cover the pillow with a towel.

3. Ask the patient to move to the side of the bed near the nurse.

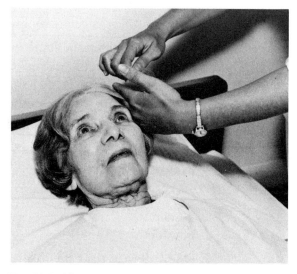

Fig. 42-1 Hold a small amount of hair near the scalp to prevent pulling.

Assist the patient in turning whenever necessary.

4. Part or section the hair. Comb with one hand between scalp and end of hair.

   This prevents pulling the hair and causing discomfort.

5. Brush carefully and thoroughly.

6. Turn the patient's head so the hair on the back of head may also be combed and brushed.

If hair is snarled, work section by section. Unsnarl, beginning near the ends and working toward scalp.

7. Complete brushing the hair; arrange attractively.

   Braiding long hair prevents snarling. Some patients may request this as part of routine evening care.

8. Clean and replace equipment.

   Each patient should have at least one comb or brush. Never use the same comb (or brush) for more than one patient.

VOCABULARY

- Define the following words:

compliment	scalp
dandruff	snarled

SUGGESTED ACTIVITY

- Visit a local drugstore and ask to see the different types of dry shampoos available. Discuss later with the instructor how to use each kind. Discuss the hazards of using both the dry and wet shampoo methods.

REVIEW

Briefly answer the following questions.

1. Give four reasons for combing and brushing the hair.

2. Describe the way to comb snarls out of the patient's hair.

3. How can the patient's hair be cleansed if the patient cannot receive a regular shampoo?

4. How can the nurse encourage patients who show no interest in combing their own hair?

5. How can the nurse prevent soiling the pillow while caring for the patient's hair?

unit 43 helping the patient to dress

OBJECTIVES

After studying this unit, the student will be able to:

- Explain how to change a patient's gown.
- Describe how the nurse can help the patient dress.
- Identify examples of conditions when a patient may need this help.

It is necessary for a patient to change clothing frequently during a hospital stay. Patients usually prefer to dress and undress themselves. However, there are times when the patient will need help and encouragement. The nurse should be there, ready to help when necessary and reduce discomfort and pain involved when changing clothing.

Dressing may be difficult for a patient who has had a stroke or is wearing a cast. Many conditions restrict range of motion or prohibit activity. The nurse must not appear hurried or impatient. Providing privacy is important when helping the patient to dress or undress.

CHANGING THE OPEN-BACK GOWN

The open-back gown is most often used in hospitals because it is easy to change. Gowns become soiled with body discharges and should be changed whenever they are wet. Although the open back makes changing easier, this feature also exposes the patient. The nurse should be sure to secure the ties at the back of the gown.

PROCEDURE

1. Obtain a clean gown and bath blanket.
2. Screen the unit and explain the procedure to the patient.
3. Place a bath blanket over the patient before removing the gown.

Prevent exposing or chilling the patient.

4. Turn the patient to a side-lying position and loosen the ties at the back of the gown.

If the patient has a sore arm, turn the patient so that arm is covered first.

5. Slip the gown off the free shoulder and take the patient's arm out of the gown sleeve.

Be sure to keep the patient covered with the bath blanket.

6. Turn the patient on the opposite side to free the gown completely.

Assist the patient to remain in the side-lying position.

7. Place the soiled gown at the foot of bed or on a chair.

Heavily soiled gowns may be wrapped in a towel.

8. Lay a clean gown over the patient and slide the bath blanket out from under the gown.

9. Slip the arm on top through the sleeve and pull the edge of the gown to the spine.

10. Turn the patient to the opposite side holding the gown in place.

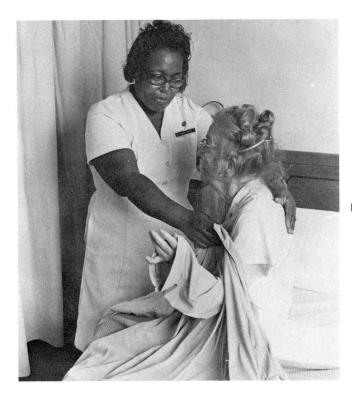

Fig. 43-1 Dress a sore or injured arm first.

Keep the edge of the gown near the spine while turning.

11. Ease the patient's other arm through the sleeve and pull the gown over the shoulder and side.

12. Bring the gown together in the back and secure the ties.

    Straighten any wrinkles in the back of the gown.

13. Assist the patient into a comfortable position. Arrange the bedcovers.

    Leave the patient in a different position from the one held prior to the gown change.

ASSISTING THE PATIENT TO DRESS

A garment which does not open in the front or back may be difficult for some patients to put on. The patient who wishes to dress in a shirt, slip, or sweater of this design may need help. The patient also may need help putting on pants or pajama bottoms. The nurse can help reduce the discomfort and fatigue that dressing may create for a patient.

PROCEDURE

1. Bring the shirt, pants, and a bath blanket to the bedside.

2. Screen the unit and explain how the garments will be put on.

    If the patient is screened well, the bath blanket may not be needed to prevent exposure.

3. Assist the patient to a sitting position, either in the bed or on the side of the bed if the patient is able.

    Do not leave the patient sitting at the side of the bed unattended.

4. To put on a shirt that does not open down the front or back, have the patient put both arms through the sleeves first.

5. Gather the bottom hem to the neckline; slip this over the patient's head.

6. Pull it down gently, first over the far shoulder and then the near shoulder.

   If one arm is sore or injured, pull the shirt down on that side first.

7. When helping with pants or pajama bottoms, gather one pant leg from the lower hem or cuff to the waist. Slip the pant leg over one foot.

8. Gather the other pant leg in the same manner, slipping it over the other foot.

9. If the patient is sitting on the side of the bed, assist him to a standing position. Pull up the pants; fasten them at the waist.

   Support the patient in the standing position.

10. If the patient is sitting in bed, help him to lie back down.

11. Ask the patient to press the heels against the bed and lift the hips. Pull the pants up as he raises his body. Fasten the pajamas at the waist.

12. To put on socks or stockings, roll the top edge down to the toe.

13. Place the patient's foot into the toe of the sock or stocking. Bring the top edge around the heel of the foot gently. Pull the sock or stocking up smoothly.

14. Assist the patient to a comfortable position and arrange the bedcovers.

VOCABULARY

- Define the following words:

  range of motion   stroke

SUGGESTED ACTIVITY

- Ask another student to role play a patient. Assume the patient is weak and has little strength in the right arm. Assist the patient into a pajama top which has no ties, only a neck opening.

REVIEW

Select the *best* answer.

1. The nurse may have to help dress the patient who has

   a. a cast
   b. suffered a stroke
   c. limited range of motion
   d. all of the above

2. If a patient has one sore arm, the nurse should

   a. keep it straight
   b. give it more exercise than the other
   c. dress it first
   d. all of the above

3. The advantage of a hospital gown over personal nightwear is that it

   a. can be changed easily
   b. exposes the patient less
   c. reminds patients of their illness
   d. is wrinkle-free

4. When putting on a shirt which does not have ties or snaps, the patient should first

   a. pull the sleeves inside out
   b. pull the shirt over the head
   c. put both arms through the sleeves
   d. none of the above

5. The weak patient who is being dressed in pajama bottoms can help by

   a. standing up in the bed
   b. lifting the hips
   c. lifting one leg at a time
   d. turning to one side

SELF-EVALUATION VII

A.   Select the *best* answer.

1.   The patient's back is washed using
    a. short, pressured strokes
    b. the heel of the hand
    c. a light, wisping motion
    d. long, firm strokes

2.   After use, the bedpan should be rinsed first with
    a. hot water
    b. cold water
    c. sterilizing solution
    d. disinfectant

3.   To promote satisfactory waste elimination, the patient should
    a. have privacy by screening the unit
    b. be left alone if the condition permits
    c. have the call signal within reach
    d. all of the above

4.   When it appears that the use of the bedpan tires the patient, the nurse should
    a. send the patient to the bathroom
    b. provide a bedside commode
    c. report this to the physician
    d. provide a high fiber diet

5.   The patient can help the nurse position a bedpan by
    a. raising the bedcovers
    b. raising the bed
    c. bending the knees
    d. raising the hips

6.   Oral hygiene
    a. aids in preventing tooth decay
    b. is refreshing
    c. stimulates the appetite
    d. all of these

7.   If the hair is badly snarled, the nurse should
    a. cut out the snarls
    b. use hair spray or dry shampoo on the hair
    c. comb, working from the ends toward the scalp
    d. comb, working from the scalp to the ends

8.   Using lemon-glycerin swabs around the mouth prevents
    a. sordes
    b. caries
    c. cavities
    d. oral paralysis

9.   The Celsius temperature for a tub bath should be in the range of
    a. 43-48°C
    b. 24-34°C
    c. 35-41°C
    d. 40-54°C

10. A nurse who observes any sign of weakness in a patient who is getting a tub bath should

    a. help the patient to get out of the tub
    b. drain the water from the tub and flash the call signal
    c. give the patient a warm drink
    d. call for help in a loud voice

B. Match the descriptions in column I with the correct terms in column II.

Column I	Column II
_____ 1. foul, brown secretions which form into crusts around the lips and teeth	a. bed bath
_____ 2. complete washing the patient receives while lying in bed	b. cold water
	c. padded tongue blade
_____ 3. prevents protein from coagulating	d. oral hygiene
_____ 4. used in giving oral hygiene to helpless patients	e. sordes
_____ 5. care of the mouth and teeth	

C. Briefly answer the following questions.

1. Name two reasons for giving a back rub.

2. Name two purposes for giving a patient oral hygiene.

3. Explain why the nurse should not leave a weak patient unattended in the tub.

4. Name three safety devices for the patient in the shower or tub.

5. Name three reasons for combing and brushing the patient's hair daily.

6. How long does a back rub usually take?

7. When giving a bed bath, the water is usually changed after washing what part of the body?

8. Why is the washcloth folded around the hand like a mitt?

9. Where are dentures stored when not in use?

10. What activities are included in morning care? List them in the order you would follow after greeting the patient.

D. Using lines and arrows, draw two diagrams showing two different strokes used to give a patient a back rub.

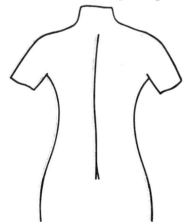 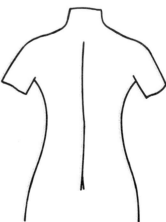

SECTION VIII ASEPTIC TECHNIQUES
unit 44 isolation procedures

OBJECTIVES

After studying this unit, the student will be able to:

- Define medical asepsis.
- Explain the care of linen, dishes, and equipment from an isolation unit.
- Define concurrent and terminal disinfection.
- Explain why specific procedures are done in the care of patients in isolation units.

Patient isolation is a method of separating a patient from other persons in a health facility. This is done when it is suspected that he has a communicable disease which can be spread to others. To prevent spread, the patient is put in a room alone; health personnel use special isolation procedures when entering or leaving the room. Isolation technique reduces the possibility of reinfection and of spreading germs through fomites. *Fomites* are inanimate items such as tissues, pencils, and silverware which carry germs from one person to another.

MEDICAL ASEPSIS

Medical asepsis is the destruction of disease-causing organisms after they leave the body. As part of medical asepsis, the nurse must use good handwashing technique. Disease is spread most easily by the hands. Doctors and other health team members often must be reminded to wash the hands when leaving the isolation unit.

Other procedures are used to achieve medical asepsis such as wearing a gown and gloves and taking special care of linen, dishes and equipment. Tasks such as bedmaking, floor sweeping and dusting require special care. Dust can carry *pathogens*, which are disease-causing organisms. Pathogens which cause respiratory disease are easily spread through inhaling room dust. Nurses and housekeeping personnel should use damp mops and cloths to clean. Using large, sweeping movements should be avoided.

Isolation technique has been simplified by the use of disposable materials. Disposable gloves, gowns, masks, and dishes are now in common use. Treatment kits also may be disposable. Kits are available for enemas, catheterizations, venipunctures or irrigations. Equipment which cannot be discarded should be securely wrapped or well scrubbed with antiseptic after use in the unit.

TAKING VITAL SIGNS

Before putting on the gown to care for the patient in an isolation unit, the nurse places a clean paper towel on the bedside table. She places her watch on it. She then puts on the gown and takes the temperature, pulse and respiration. After wiping the thermometer it is kept in antiseptic solution in the unit. The thermometer is placed in this solution after each use. The nurse removes the gown and thoroughly washes her hands. The watch can be put back on just before the nurse leaves the room.

CARE OF LINEN

Linen taken from an isolation unit is a hazard to those handling it. To reduce the risk of disease spread, the linen is sent to the laundry in a special bag. This bag has the word, *Isolation* imprinted on it, or it may have a colored stripe around it. Use of a special bag alerts all personnel to the fact that the contents are contaminated.

Contaminated items are those which have been exposed to pathogens. The isolation bag fits around the contaminated bag which contains the linen. This is called *double-bagging*. When properly closed, the isolation bag remains "clean" on the outside.

PROCEDURE

1. Assemble supplies:

   Gown
   Gloves
   Mask
   Clean laundry bag (colored or labeled *Isolation*)
   Regular laundry bag

2. Ask another health team member to stand outside the patient's room and hold the clean laundry bag.

   The nurse outside the door does not become contaminated if linen is bagged correctly.

3. Dress in the gown, gloves and mask and enter the isolation room.

4. Collect soiled linen and place in a regular laundry bag.

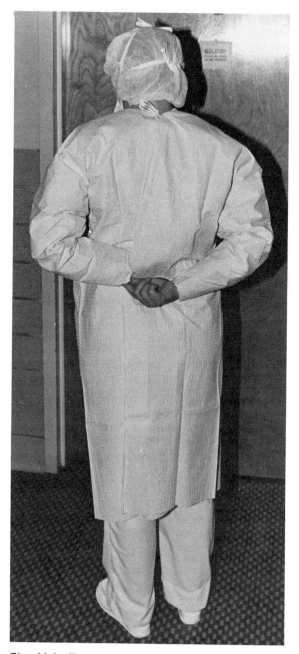

Fig. 44-1 To enter some isolation rooms, the nurse may need the complete protection of a mask, cap, gown and gloves.

5. Tie the bag tightly and carry the bag to the doorway.

   Do not drag the bag across the floor. This raises dust and spreads germs.

6. Ask the clean nurse outside the door to hold the clean bag open.

The clean nurse should cuff the top of the bag, keeping both hands under the cuff, figure 44-2.

7. Remain in the isolation room and place the filled laundry bag into the clean bag which is being held outside the room.

   Do not touch the outside of the clean bag. If necessary, the inside may be touched.

8. Ask the clean nurse to close the clean bag around the contaminated one.

   The clean nurse should touch only the outside of the clean bag.

9. Ask the clean nurse to label the isolation bag, if necessary, and to take it to the laundry chute.

10. Remove the gown, mask and gloves before leaving the isolation unit.

CARE OF DISHES

The dishes used by a patient with an infectious disease are contaminated. For this reason, they must be handled carefully. Leftover food should remain on the dishes. Nondisposable dishes must be tightly sealed in a plastic bag before they are taken from the room. The bag should be tied securely with clean hands. This prevents the outside of the bag from becoming contaminated. Dishes should be double-bagged in the same way linen is. All bags containing contaminated material should be labeled *Isolation*. Nondisposable dishes must be soaked in hot water and disinfectant. They must be kept separate from other patients' dishes. In most facilities dishes are disinfected in the central supply department.

Disposable cups, dishes and flatware are in general use. They are discarded along with leftover food wastes in a plastic bag. The bag must be tightly sealed and double-bagged. The outside should be labeled *Isolation*.

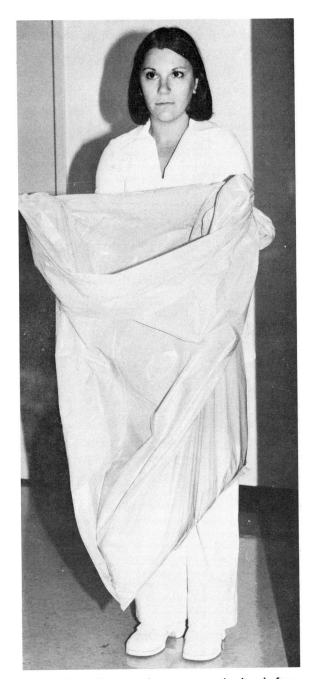

Fig. 44-2 Cuffing the bag protects the hands from contamination.

DISPOSING OF WASTES OR BODY DISCHARGES

Pathogenic organisms often exist in urine, feces, vomitus, sputum or wound drainage. Most health facilities are served by a sewage treatment plant which disinfects any matter disposed of in the toilet or hopper. Facilities not equipped in this way can disinfect wastes by using chlorinated lime. The lime is spread over the contaminated matter and allowed to remain for four hours. Secretions or wastes can then be disposed of safely.

CONCURRENT DISINFECTION OF EQUIPMENT

Concurrent daily disinfection frees articles from pathogens so the patient can safely reuse them within the room. Certain pathogens are difficult to destroy. Those such as the hepatitis virus, tubercle bacillus, and tetanus bacillus spores require a special disinfection process. Many hospitals use only disposable equipment for isolation patients.

TERMINAL DISINFECTION

Terminal disinfection is the thorough cleaning of the room and all equipment after the patient has left. It includes autoclaving all equipment, airing the room and laundering linen and blankets. In an isolation room, the floors and walls are disinfected. Disposable articles are wrapped in paper and then placed in a paper bag. The bag and its contents can then be burned.

VOCABULARY

- Define the following words:

chlorinated lime	fomite	reinfecting
communicable	hepatitis virus	spore
disposable	infectious	tetanus bacillus
double-bagged	irrigation	

SUGGESTED ACTIVITIES

- Investigate the methods of disinfecting excreta in communities where a municipal sewage disposal system is in operation.

- Practice taking temperature, pulse and respiration, using the adaptations necessary for the isolation unit. Students should evaluate each other's skill.

- Demonstrate the handling of soiled linen from an isolation unit.

REVIEW

Briefly answer the following questions.

1. How should secretions and wastes from a patient in an isolation unit be disinfected in facilities which have no municipal sewage disposal system?

2. How should nondisposable dishes from an isolation unit be treated before being returned to the kitchen?

3. What is terminal disinfection?

4. What is concurrent disinfection?

5. Name three pathogens which are especially difficult to destroy.

6. What is double-bagging?

7. What is a fomite?

8. Why are two persons needed to care for soiled linen from the isolation room?

9. What is the reason for placing a patient in isolation?

10. Name three items which must be worn when working in an isolation room.

unit 45 sterile glove technique

OBJECTIVES

After studying this unit, the student will be able to:

- Name two procedures that require the use of sterile gloves.
- Explain the procedure used to put on sterile gloves.
- Describe how to remove gloves without contaminating the hands.

The nurse may often be required to wear sterile gloves. Performing or assisting with sterile procedures such as dressing changes or catheterizations require the use of sterile gloves. Major or minor surgical procedures always require that assistants wear sterile gloves. Nurses can use gloves to protect the patients and themselves from transmitting disease.

PROCEDURE

1. Obtain a package of sterile gloves.

   Gloves are prepowdered or come with a powder pack to ease slipping them on.

2. Wash and dry hands thoroughly.

   Using gloves should never substitute for good handwashing. Hands that are thoroughly dry make the gloves easier to put on.

3. Open package, grasping only the corners.

   Do not touch the inside of the wrapper.

4. Apply powder to hands from powder pack if needed.

   Do not hold hands over sterile gloves while powdering.

5. Lift and hold one-half of the wrapper. With the other hand, remove one glove, touching only the top of the cuff.

6. Slip hand into glove and pull glove over hand carefully.

   Hold glove by inside of cuff. Do not adjust the fingers of the glove by touching the outside.

7. Lift up other side of wrapper with bare hand. Remove other glove by placing gloved fingers under the cuff.

   Do not contaminate gloved hand.

8. Pull glove over bare hand by grasping the cuff.

9. Turn out both cuffs.

   Touch only the sterile outer surface of the gloves with gloved hands. After gloves have been put on, touch only sterile surfaces with gloves. If gloves become contaminated, remove them and put on another pair.

REMOVING GLOVES

The nurse must be as careful in removing gloves as in putting them on. The technique used to remove them is for the nurse's protection. Contaminated hands create a hazard for the nurse and the patients whom the nurse may contact.

PROCEDURE

1. If nondisposable gloves are used, they must be rinsed under cold running water before being removed.

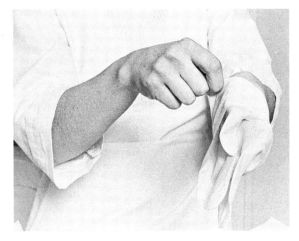

(A) Put on one glove touching only the top of the folded cuff.

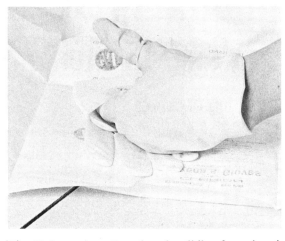

(B) Pick up the other glove by sliding four gloved fingers under the cuff.

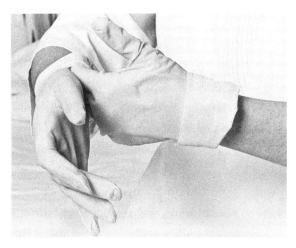

(C) Fit the fingers into the glove carefully.

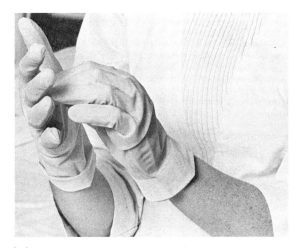

(D) Adjust the fingers and cuffs without touching the bare skin.

Fig. 45-1 Putting on sterile gloves.

This prevents organic matter from adhering to surface during cleaning.

2. Grasp the first glove on the outside of the cuff. Pull the glove over the hand, wrong side out.

The contaminated surface of the glove is turned inside.

3. Grasp second glove from the inside using the bare fingers. Remove glove by pulling it over hand, wrong side out.

4. After gloves have been removed, do not touch equipment or instruments which have been contaminated.

SUGGESTED ACTIVITY

- Practice putting on and taking off gloves. Avoid contamination of gloves when putting them on and avoid contamination of hands when taking the gloves off.

REVIEW

Briefly answer the following questions.

1. Name two sterile procedures which require the use of sterile gloves.

2. Why should the hands be dry and powdered before putting on gloves?

3. Explain the procedure for removing contaminated gloves.

4. Why should nondisposable gloves be rinsed with cold water before removing them?

5. Where does the nurse grasp the package of sterile gloves to open it?

unit 46 sterile dressings

OBJECTIVES

After studying this unit, the student will be able to:

- Explain how to prepare a sterile field for dressing change.
- Describe the technique used to clean a wound.
- Identify reasons behind each procedural step.

One of the most effective ways the body defends itself from disease is by maintaining healthy unbroken skin. A wound or incision will break down this natural defense. Therefore, any break in the skin must be treated to prevent organisms from entering. One means of protection is by the use of sterile dressings. The word *sterile* means free from all microorganisms (germs). A *sterile dressing* is material that has been treated so that it is germfree and may be applied to a wound.

To apply a sterile dressing, sterile technique must be used in order not to contaminate the dressing while putting it on. Part of using sterile technique is setting up a sterile field. A *sterile field* is a work area where sterile supplies can be placed without becoming contaminated.

The nurse can contaminate a sterile field or area in the following ways:

- reaching over or passing through the sterile field
- dropping anything which is not sterile into the area (unsterile dressings or glove powder)
- splashing water or any fluid (even sterile fluids) into the area
- raising dust; or speaking unmasked or through a moist mask

Sterile technique is used to achieve surgical asepsis. *Surgical asepsis* is the destruction of organisms before they enter the body.

PREPARING A STERILE FIELD FOR A DRESSING CHANGE

The nurse may change the dressing or help another team member to do so. In either case, using surgical aseptic technique is necessary. Good handwashing technique always precedes setting up the sterile field. Gathering supplies and placing them around the bedside must be done before putting on sterile gloves. The nurse can not handle unsterile items once the dressing change is in process.

PROCEDURE

1. Assemble equipment:
   Dressing tray containing:
   Gauze sponges
   Gloves
   Sterile towel
   Sterile basin
   Solution as ordered
   Abdominal pads
   Adhesive tape or binder

   Place a paper bag or basin at the foot of the bed to receive soiled dressings when they have been removed.

   Size and number of gauze sponges and abdominal pads will vary.

2. Greet patient and explain procedure.

3. Screen the unit and drape the patient to expose only the area to be dressed.

4. Organize supplies and set up the sterile field.

5. If sterile dressings are in separate packages, open them but do not touch the inside.

   Do not contaminate sterile dressings with ungloved hands.

6. Open the sterile towel and place it on the bed near the wound area.

   Touch only the corners of the towel to set up a sterile field.

7. Place dressings on sterile towel, figure 46-1.

   The field must remain sterile. Be sure not to reach over the field when dropping the sponges.

8. Pour antiseptic solution into a basin.

9. Remove the old dressing by loosening the outside edges of the tape first.

   Always pull toward the wound to avoid putting strain on healing tissue.

10. If the dressing sticks to the wound, soak it off with hydrogen peroxide, sterile water, or saline.

    Check the doctor's order to see whether he prefers a particular solution.

11. Observe the soiled dressing; note the amount, color, and nature of the drainage.

    Record observations on the chart at the end of the procedure.

12. Discard the soiled dressing in the basin at the foot of the bed.

    Do not bring the dressings near the sterile field.

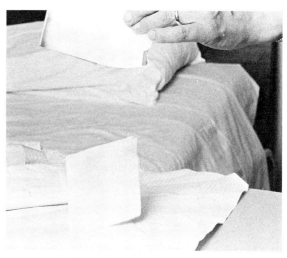

Fig. 46-1 Carefully drop sterile dressings on to the sterile towel. Do not reach over the sterile field.

CLEANSING THE WOUND AND APPLYING THE DRESSING

The doctor may wish to change a patient's dressing but often asks the nurse to do it. The nurse should learn how to assist the doctor and how to perform the procedure. Both require the use of good handwashing and maintenance of a sterile field.

ASSISTING THE DOCTOR WITH A DRESSING CHANGE

When assisting the doctor, the nurse may remove the old dressing but saves it for the doctor to view. The main task of the nurse is to open the packages of sterile gloves, gauze and dressings, as the doctor needs them. The doctor can then change the dressing easily without contaminating the sterile gloves. To keep the items sterile, the nurse must not touch the inside of any packages. If the supplies have been prepared and organized, the sterile field is not likely to become contaminated.

CHANGING A DRESSING

Minor wounds are usually dressed by the nurse. However, even minor wounds can become infected so the nurse must use sterile technique. Preparation of the sterile field and gathering of supplies should be done before putting on the sterile gloves.

PROCEDURE

1. Check to see that the needed supplies are within reach.

   Review the list provided earlier in this unit.

2. Put on sterile gloves in order to clean the wound.

3. Moisten the gauze squares in the antiseptic solution ordered.

   Do not drip over the sterile field.

4. Clean the surface of the wound with a single stroke.

   Do not go back over the same area with the same gauze or the area will be contaminated.

5. Discard the gauze sponge in the basin where the soiled dressing was placed.

6. Using a clean gauze sponge, clean the skin around the wound. Start at the wound and work outward.

   Do not go back over the wound.

7. Repeat the procedure until the area has been cleaned.

8. Observe the wound and apply medication if ordered.

   Observe for pus, redness, and evidence of scab formation.

9. Dry the wound area with sterile gauze and discard in the basin at the foot of the bed.

   Pat the area dry; do not rub.

10. Place the new sterile dressing on the wound.

    Be sure to completely cover the wound.

11. Secure the dressings with adhesive tape, nonallergic tape, or a binder.

    Paper tape is the least irritating to the skin but is not as strong.

12. Remove the gloves, turning them inside out.

13. Clean up the bedside area and replace used items.

14. Record observations made about the wound. Notify the charge nurse if they are unusual.

VOCABULARY

- Define the following words:

| forceps | nonallergic | contaminate |
| hydrogen peroxide | saline | sterile |

SUGGESTED ACTIVITIES

- Obtain a dressing, towel, basin and forceps. Practice transferring a dressing from the package to the towel as if maintaining a sterile field.

- Practice opening sterile packages of gauze sponges and gloves. Do not contaminate the gauze, the gloves, or the inside of the packages.

- Demonstrate applying a sterile dressing to an arm or hand.

REVIEW

Select the *best* answer.

1. Antiseptic solution is used on a wound to

    a. sterilize the wound
    b. clean the wound
    c. free the old dressing
    d. keep the new dressing from sticking to the wound

2. A natural defense which protects the body from disease is

    a. the skin
    b. a bandage dressing
    c. medication ordered by the doctor
    d. use of sterile technique

3. Sterile technique is used to apply a sterile dressing in order to

    a. use fewer supplies
    b. reduce cleanup time after the procedure
    c. discipline health team members to be neat
    d. avoid contaminating the dressing

4. The sterile field may be contaminated by

    a. touching the sterile towel with the sterile forceps
    b. touching the outside of a package with ungloved hands
    c. splashing antiseptic into the area
    d. dropping a sterile dressing on the sterile towel

5. Tape is pulled off toward the wound rather than away from it because

    a. this lessens the strain on the wound
    b. the tape loosens more easily
    c. the dressing may tear otherwise
    d. the wound must remain sterile

6. The dressing may be soaked off the wound with

    a. hydrogen peroxide
    b. cool tap water
    c. warm tap water
    d. none of the above

7. The main concern of the nurse who is helping a doctor with a dressing change is to

    a. please the doctor
    b. calm the patient
    c. prevent possible contamination
    d. learn how to change dressings

8. When opening a package of sterile gauze sponges for the doctor, the nurse should

    a. wear sterile gloves
    b. discard the package and hold the dressings
    c. place the package on the sterile towel
    d. touch only the outside of the package

9. To clean the area of the wound, the moistened gauze sponge should be moved

   a. toward the wound   c. across the wound
   b. away from the wound   d. none of the above

10. Paper tape is sometimes used on the skin instead of adhesive tape because it

   a. is stronger   c. is sterile
   b. is less irritating   d. adheres better

unit 47 applying binders

OBJECTIVES

After studying this unit, the student will be able to:

- Name four reasons for using binders.
- Identify the types of binders and the function of each.
- Describe the method used to apply each binder to the body.

A binder is a wide band of muslin or heavy cotton material; it may have one or more tails. Binders are used to provide body support, hold dressings in place, apply pressure, or limit motion of a body part. The nurse should check the order before putting a binder on a patient. Knowing the purpose for the binder is necessary in order to put it on correctly. Binders must be applied smoothly. Wrinkles can cause irritation; this is uncomfortable and may lead to decubiti.

APPLYING THE STRAIGHT BINDER TO THE ABDOMEN

The straight binder must be applied to fit the contour of the body. If necessary, small tucks can be made to improve the fit. Abdominal binders are usually applied for support. Therefore, the nurse should apply the binder snugly. It should exert slight pressure around the abdomen.

PROCEDURE

1. Assemble equipment:

   Straight binder   Safety pins
2. Greet the patient and explain the procedure.
3. Screen the unit.
4. Fanfold the top bedcovers to pubic area and lift the patient's gown to expose the abdomen.
5. Help the patient to move to the near side of bed, in a back-lying position.
6. Ask the patient to flex the knees, press down on the heels, and lift the hips.

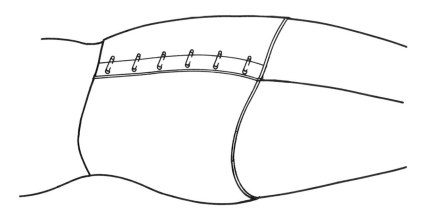

Fig. 47-1 The straight binder can be applied to the chest or abdomen.

7. Fold the binder to determine where the center will be. Then slide the binder under the patient's lower back. Center the binder and place the lower edge just beyond the curves of the buttocks.

Place the binder so that it will not interfere with walking or use of the bedpan.

8. Bring each end of the binder up over the patient's abdomen; overlap, and pin them together in the center. Place the pins no more than 5 cm (2 inches) apart.

Apply pins in a straight line. Place your fingers under the binder to protect the patient when pinning.

9. Position the patient comfortably. Rearrange gown and replace top bedcovers.

10. Record unusual observations or any changes in the patient's condition.

APPLYING A STRAIGHT BINDER TO THE BREASTS

Applying a binder around the breasts provides support. Engorged breasts during lactation may require extra support. A woman who has had breast surgery may also receive comfort from a breast binder.

PROCEDURE

1. Obtain the binder and pins.

2. Explain the procedure to the patient and prepare the unit.

3. Help the patient to a back-lying position. Fanfold the top bedcovers to the waist.

4. Untie the gown and ask the patient to slip both arms out of the sleeves.

5. Allow the gown to rest on top of the patient to act as a drape.

6. Help the patient to turn on the side.

7. Place the binder at the back so the top edge lines up with the axillae (underarms).

8. Help the patient to roll back onto the binder.

Straighten the binder so it is smooth and in position.

9. Bring the ends of the binder up over the patient's chest. There should be a 2-inch overlap.

10. With your hands on the binder, raise breasts up and toward the center. Ask patient to hold breasts in position if she is able.

11. Starting in the center of the binder, pin the overlap. Pin downward to the bottom edge. Return to the center and pin toward the top edge.

Pin the binder snugly enough to support the breasts well.

12. Bring the straps of the binder up over each shoulder. Pin the ends to the front of the binder.

13. Help the patient back into the gown and position comfortably.

14. Record the procedure and report unusual observations.

APPLYING A T-BINDER

A T-binder is used to hold rectal or perineal dressings in place. A double T-binder is used by males to hold dressings or support the scrotum. The belt is pinned around the waist. The tails are passed between the legs and pinned to the belt, figure 47-2.

PROCEDURE

1. Obtain a single or double T-binder and the safety pins.

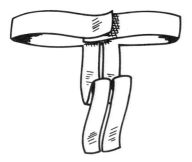
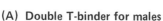
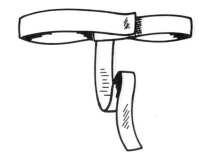

(A) Double T-binder for males   (B) T-binder for females

Fig. 47-2 T-binders fit easily around the waist and between the legs.

2. Explain the procedure to the patient and screen the unit.

3. Fanfold the bedcovers to the pubic area. Help the patient to assume a back-lying position.

4. Ask the patient to lift the hips. Place center of the binder at the patient's spine.

5. Adjust straps to fit waist. Secure with safety pin at the center of the waist.

    Make sure there are no twists or wrinkles.

6. Bring T-strap up between legs to waist. Fasten strap to waistband with pin.

7. If a double T-binder is applied, bring one strap up along each side of the genitals and fasten to the belt with pins.

    Ask the patient if the binder is comfortable. If dressings are present, be sure they are in place.

8. Help the patient into a comfortable position.

9. Rearrange the gown and replace the top bedcovers.

10. Report and record unusual observations.

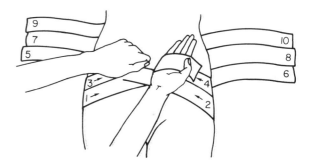

Fig. 47-3 Each tail of the scultetus binder is applied upward in an overlapping fashion.

APPLYING THE SCULTETUS BINDER

Scultetus binders are also called many-tailed binders. They are used to support the abdomen or hold dressings in place. They can also be applied to the chest for the same reasons. There may be four to ten tails which wrap around the body, the bottom tails are applied first. A tail is brought up from each side and lapped in oblique placement, figure 47-3. The last two tails are crossed downward, diagonally, to the lower edge of the binder and are secured with safety pins.

PROCEDURE

1. Obtain the scultetus binder and safety pins.

2. Explain the procedure and screen the unit.

3. Fanfold the top bedcovers to the pubic area and lift the patient's gown to expose the abdomen.

4. Ask the patient to assume a back-lying position and to lift the hips.

   Assist the patient if necessary.

5. Slide the binder under the lower back. Center the binder under the spine and place the lower edge at the base of the spine.

   Make sure that the binder is not placed so low that it will interfere with the use of the bedpan. Be sure the part of the binder under the patient is straight before proceeding with application of the tails.

6. Beginning at the bottom edge, bring tails up one by one over the abdomen.

   Alternate sides. The tails should cross diagonally at the center of the abdomen. Tuck in each end securely.

   Make sure binder fits snugly. There should be no wrinkles. Ends should not be tucked in over the hip bones.

7. Cross the last two tails diagonally across the abdomen from the top of the binder and pin at the lower edge.

   Place fingers under binder when pinning to protect patient.

8. Position the patient comfortably. Rearrange gown and replace the top bedcovers.

9. Record the procedure and report any unusual observations.

VOCABULARY

- Define the following words:

contour	muslin	pubic
engorged	oblique	scrotum
lactation	overlap	scultetus

SUGGESTED ACTIVITY

- Ask the instructor to help locate the various binders. Using a mannequin, practice applying the binders.

REVIEW

A. Select the *best* answer.

1. The binder that is used to hold rectal or perineal dressings in place is the
   a. T-binder
   b. straight binder
   c. abdominal binder
   d. scultetus binder

2. The type of binder that is usually applied for support is the
   a. T-binder
   b. straight binder
   c. double T-binder
   d. none of these

3. When the straight binder is applied to the abdomen, it is

   a. centered under the patient's spine
   b. placed so the lower edge is just beyond the buttocks
   c. slid under the patient's lower back
   d. all of the above

4. A T-binder is placed

   a. under the base of the patient's spine
   b. so the lower edge is just beyond the buttocks
   c. so the top edge lines up with the axillae
   d. none of the above

5. A scultetus binder may be

   a. used to support the abdomen
   b. used to hold dressings against the abdomen
   c. placed under the patient's lower back
   d. all of the above

B. Briefly answer the following questions.

1. List four purposes of binders.

2. Why should the nurse know the reason why a binder has been ordered?

3. Why should the nurse be particularly careful not to wrinkle or twist a binder when applying it?

4. What binder(s) fit between the legs?

5. State two reasons why a woman may need a breast binder.

SELF-EVALUATION VIII

A. Match the definitions in column I with the correct terms in column II. Insert the letter before the definitions.

Column I

_____ 1. destruction of organisms before they enter the body

_____ 2. state in which a disease may spread to others

_____ 3. work area where sterile supplies can be placed

_____ 4. destruction of disease-causing organisms after they leave the body

_____ 5. state in which an item has been exposed to pathogens

_____ 6. disease-causing organisms

Column II

a. contaminated
b. communicable
c. medical asepsis
d. pathogens
e. sterile field
f. surgical asepsis

B. Select the *best* answer.

1. Using isolation procedures is an example of

    a. medical asepsis
    b. surgical asepsis
    c. personal hygiene
    d. maintaining a sterile field

2. Surgical asepsis includes

    a. preventing infection
    b. putting on sterile gloves
    c. establishing a sterile field
    d. all of the above

3. In caring for linen from an isolation unit

    a. the outside of the colored or labeled laundry bag is considered contaminated
    b. the outside of the laundry bag in the isolation room is considered contaminated
    c. linen should be soaked in antiseptic solution before placing it in laundry chute
    d. no special care is needed

4. One of the most effective natural body defenses against disease is

    a. iodine
    b. unbroken skin
    c. vitamin C
    d. handwashing

5. Binders are applied

   a. to give support and limit motion
   b. to hold dressings in place
   c. to apply pressure
   d. all of the above

6. Excreta from a patient with a communicable disease

   a. should all be soaked in 5% solution of cresol
   b. should be burned
   c. requires no special treatment if there is a municipal sewage system
   d. should be deodorized

7. Rinsing nondisposable gloves under cold water before taking them off

   a. prevents contamination of nurse's hands
   b. prevents organic matter from adhering to the gloves
   c. kills pathogens
   d. is not necessary

8. A patient who is put on *Isolation* has a disease which is

   a. respiratory   c. nonpathogenic
   b. contaminated   d. communicable

9. Pathogens are less likely to spread if the patient's room is cleaned with a

   a. damp mop   c. sterile towel
   b. small dry cloth   d. broom

10. Terminal disinfection is necessary

    a. as a daily isolation procedure
    b. only with disposable items
    c. after the patient vacates the isolation room
    d. only after the nurse leaves the isolation room

11. Sterile gloves are worn to

    a. protect the patient
    b. protect the nurse
    c. prevent unnecessary contamination
    d. all of the above

12. A sterile towel is contaminated when touched by

    a. a sterile dressing   c. sterile forceps
    b. a dressing package   d. the doctor's sterile gloves

13. The double T-binder may be applied in order to

    a. support the male genitalia   c. apply pressure to the buttocks
    b. hold abdominal dressings   d. tighten the waist

14. The breasts can be supported by application of a

    a. scultetus binder   c. double T-binder
    b. T-binder   d. straight binder

15. When taking a sterile glove from the package, the nurse picks it up by the

    a. glove fingers   c. top of the folded cuff
    b. outside of the cuff   d. thumb of the glove

16. Disposable items used in the isolation room include

    a. mask, gown, gloves   c. catheterization kits
    b. dishes   d. all of the above

SECTION IX APPLICATIONS OF HEAT AND COLD

unit 48 ice bags and cold packs

OBJECTIVES

After studying this unit, the student will be able to:

- State the effects of cold upon the body.
- Describe how to prepare and apply an ice bag.
- Identify safety precautions used when applying cold to the body.
- Compare the advantages of dry and moist cold.

Before administering local application of cold, the nurse should know the effects it has on the body. Applying an ice bag can damage the body tissues if done incorrectly. The nurse should also know the purpose of the cold treatment. In order to be sure that the desirable effect is obtained, the nurse must understand why the patient needs the treatment.

PHYSIOLOGICAL EFFECTS

The body responds to the application of cold by shivering and forming gooseflesh. Perspiration also decreases and the skin becomes pale. If the cold treatment is prolonged, the skin becomes red and the surface temperature of the skin increases. The rate of respiration and the pulse rate decrease. Perspiration increases and the patient becomes relaxed. Comfort, similar to that produced by the prolonged application of heat, is experienced with cold.

These effects occur because cold decreases the supply of blood to an area. Cold contracts the blood vessels causing *vasoconstriction* (narrowing of the blood vessels). Because of the reduced blood supply, both in-

flammation and hemorrhage can be slowed. Reduced blood flow can prevent *ecchymosis* (bruise marks). General application of cold may produce sedation or reduce body temperature.

TYPES OF COLD APPLICATIONS

There are two kinds of cold which are applied to parts of the body. They are known as dry cold and moist cold. Moist cold is applied by use of compresses or cold packs. Moist cold is more penetrating than dry cold. Dry cold is applied by the use of the ice bag, ice cap, or collar. An ice bag or cap is a rubber or plastic container made in many sizes to apply to various parts of the body. The ice collar is narrow and suitable for use on the neck or on a small area. Both are used frequently as a method of applying dry cold.

Commercially prepared cold packs may be used instead of ice bags. They maintain a constant degree of cold and eliminate the need for frequent refilling. These packs usually stay cold up to 60 minutes. However, this depends upon the size of the pack and the chemical it contains. When the cold pack melts, it must be wiped clean and returned to the freezer. Another way to maintain constant temperature is through the use of a special water-filled pad (aquamatic pad). The water in the pad is chilled, and the temperature is controlled by a gauge on a separate, electric control unit. Both of these methods maintain a constant cold temperature without requiring any refilling. Because of this, it is possible to forget to check the patient frequently. CAUTION: Whatever method is used, the nurse should check the patient's condition and examine the area of application every fifteen minutes.

SAFETY PRECAUTIONS

Any ice bag, collar, pack, or water-filled pad must be covered before it touches the skin. Skin can be damaged from direct exposure to cold. Each patient's reaction to cold is different. Therefore, the nurse should not leave a patient alone for a long period. The patient should be checked every 15 minutes. More frequent checks should be made with infants, young children, the aged, or patients who have poor circulation. Because the effects of cold can cause a major change in the patient's condition a written order from the doctor is required for its use.

PROCEDURE

1. Assemble and prepare equipment in utility room:

   Ice bag, cap or collar
   Cover
   Paper towels
   Ice cubes or crushed ice
   Ice scoop or spoon

   Crushed ice will fill the bag in a way that will fit body parts more satisfactorily than cubes.

2. If large ice cubes are used, break or crush them.

3. Fill the ice bag half-full, using an ice scoop or large spoon.

   This allows the bag to conform to body better. It also prevents the bag from becoming too heavy.

4. Expel air by resting the ice bag flat on the table. Put the top in place but do not screw it on. Squeeze the bag until air has been removed.

5. Screw top on securely.

   Bag will not conform to body contours if there is air in it.

6. Test for leakage.

7. Wipe the top and the sides dry with a paper towel.

8. Place a cover around the ice bag.

   Be sure the entire surface area is covered. Never permit rubber or plastic to touch patient's skin.

9. Greet patient and explain procedure.

10. Take equipment to bedside on tray.

11. Apply the bag with the cap (metal or plastic top) facing away from the patient, figure 48-1.

    Remain with the patient for a few minutes to observe the body's reaction to the treatment.

12. Refill the bag for prolonged cold treatments.

    Check skin area with each application. Check the doctor's order for the prescribed length of the treatment.

13. If skin becomes discolored, or if patient reports the skin is numb, remove the ice bag and report to the supervising nurse.

    Prolonged use of cold can damage tissue and, therefore, must be discontinued at regular intervals.

14. When the ice bag is removed, wash it with soap and water; let it drain and allow to dry. Screw on the top when it is dry.

    Some air is left in the ice bag to prevent sides from sticking together.

15. If a reusable cold pack was used, wash it thoroughly with soap and water and return to the freezer.

    This prevents cross-infection.

16. Record the time the ice bag was applied and the length of the treatment. Note any unusual observations which result from the treatment. Report the results.

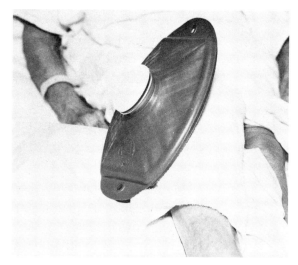

Fig. 48-1 The cap on the ice bag should face away from the patient.

VOCABULARY

- Define the following words:

  cross-infection   inflammation   vasoconstriction
  ecchymosis   penetrating   hypothermia
  gooseflesh   perspiration

SUGGESTED ACTIVITY

- Obtain an ice bag or ice collar. Practice filling it and expelling the air. Examine the cover closely and determine how well it protects the patient's skin.

REVIEW

Select the *best* answer.

1. One effect cold has upon the body is to

   a. cause vasoconstriction
   b. increase blood flow to a local area
   c. increase body temperature overall
   d. cause ecchymosis

2. Cold controls hemorrhage because

   a. bacteria are inhibited   c. blood supply is reduced
   b. circulation is cut off   d. blood vessels are dilated

3. The half-full ice bag

   a. slides off the body easier   c. becomes heavier as the ice melts
   b. conforms to the body better   d. should be left uncapped

217

4. Air is expelled from the ice bag to
   a. make the bag more flexible
   b. reduce extra weight
   c. allow the cover to fit better
   d. delay the melting of the ice

5. One difference between dry and moist cold is that
   a. dry cold is more effective
   b. moist cold is more penetrating
   c. dry cold applications can remain uncovered
   d. dry cold treatments need no attention

6. The advantage of a commercially prepared cold pack is that it
   a. maintains a constant degree of cold
   b. eliminates the need for frequent refilling
   c. stays cold up to 60 minutes
   d. all of the above

7. The advantage in using an aquamatic pad is that it
   a. maintains a constant temperature
   b. uses crushed ice
   c. can be left on indefinitely
   d. all of the above

8. Three types of patients who need to be checked more often when receiving cold treatments are
   a. infants, middle-aged women, and the elderly
   b. infants, young children, and the aged
   c. heart patients, preoperative patients, and cancer patients
   d. teenage mothers, young children, and women in menopause

9. Commercially prepared cold packs and aquamatic pads may be dangerous if
   a. they are covered
   b. the patient is not checked every 15 minutes
   c. they are not refilled frequently
   d. they do not follow the body contour

10. Safety precautions which must be followed whenever cold is applied to a patient include
    a. cover the bag or pad so it does not touch the skin
    b. check the patient's condition every 15 minutes
    c. apply cold only upon written orders from the doctor
    d. all of the above

unit 49 the hot water bag

OBJECTIVES

After studying this unit, the student will be able to:

- Explain how the application of heat affects the body.
- Name three reasons for applying heat.
- List five types of patients that are likely to be sensitive to heat.
- Describe the procedure used for applying a hot water bag.
- Identify safety precautions to be used when applying heat.

The nurse who is applying heat must use great care since heat can burn the patient. Hot applications of any type are used only when ordered by a doctor.

PHYSIOLOGICAL EFFECTS

Heat may be applied to reduce swelling, relax muscles, or promote wound healing. When heat is applied, the body reacts soon after treatment is started. Heat causes *vasodilation* (expansion of the blood vessels). Heat also increases circulation of the blood and lymph. The increased flow reduces fluid buildup in one area and thus reduces swelling. Increased circulation also brings nutrients to the area for wound healing. The increased activity causes a rise in tissue metabolism; this also promotes healing. Although treatments of long duration (time) help muscles relax, excessive heat may cause local edema (swelling).

KINDS OF HOT APPLICATIONS

The doctor may prescribe either dry heat or moist heat. Dry heat is applied by means of a hot water bag, electric heating pads, or a heat lamp. Moist heat will be discussed in units 52 through 54.

SAFETY PRECAUTIONS

Unfortunately, many patients have been burned through use of intense heat. Great care must be taken not to burn the patient. Before preparing the hot water bag, the nurse should check to be sure that the doctor has ordered it, and that she is applying it to the right patient.

Sensitivity to heat varies with each person. Those persons with light skin and and those with poor circulation must be watched carefully. Infants, young children, and the elderly are also more sensitive to heat than others. A pad, towel, or hot water bag cover should always lie between the patient's skin and the bag. The temperature of the water to be used depends on a number of factors: (1) the condition of the skin, (2) size of the area being treated, (3) length of the treatment, and (4) condition of the patient.

PROCEDURE

1. Assemble and prepare equipment in utility room:

   Hot water bag
   Container for hot water
   Paper towel
   Cover
   Bath thermometer

2. Fill container with water and test for the correct temperature. The range is about 105-125°F (41-52°C).

Use a bath thermometer to check the water temperature. **Check the doctor's order for a requested temperature guide.**

3. Fill hot water bag 1/3 to 1/2 full.

   This avoids applying unnecessary weight and helps the bag conform to the body.

4. Expel air by placing hot water bag flat on a surface and holding the neck of bag upright. When the water reaches the neck, screw on the top.

   This allows the bag to conform to body contours.

5. Wipe hot water bag dry with paper towels and turn bag upside down to check for leakage.

6. Place cover on hot water bag.

   Patient's skin must not come in contact with rubber or plastic.

7. Explain the procedure and take equipment to the bedside.

8. Apply to the affected area as ordered.

   CAUTION: Never allow a patient to lie on the hot water bag. The patient's body heat is added to that already being released by the hot water bag and severe burns may result.

9. Check the patient's condition at least every fifteen minutes.

10. Refill the bag as necessary.

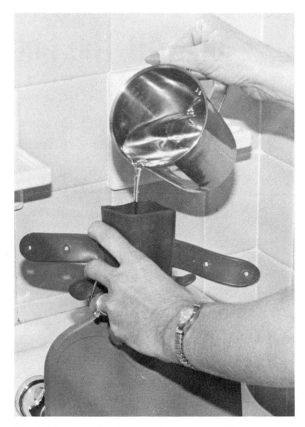

Fig. 49-1 Water in the container is tested for temperature before being poured into the bag.

Check the condition of skin before refilling the bag. Report any unusual observations to the supervising nurse.

11. Clean and replace equipment according to hospital policy. Place cover in laundry hamper.

12. Record time and length of the treatment. Record any unusual observations.

VOCABULARY

- Define the following words:

  contour   metabolism

SUGGESTED ACTIVITIES

- Obtain a hot water bag and practice filling it and closing it properly. Refer to the guidelines in this unit.

• Find a container and fill it with water. Test the temperature of the water until you obtain a reading of 105°F (41°C). Fill a hot water bag, and after covering it, place it against your arm or abdomen. Repeat the procedure using water 125°F (52°C). Decide which temperature is most comfortable for you. Are some areas of the body more heat sensitive than others?

REVIEW

Briefly answer the following questions.

1. List five types of patients who are most likely to be sensitive to heat.

2. Name four factors that determine the temperature of the water used for a heat application.

3. List three reasons for the use of the hot water bag.

4. What is the temperature range for water used to fill a hot water bag? Give the readings in both Fahrenheit and Celsius.

5. How does the application of heat affect the blood vessels?

unit 50 the electric heating pad

OBJECTIVES

After studying this unit, the student will be able to:

- State the advantages of using an electric heating pad.
- List safety precautions for use of an electric heating pad.
- Describe the procedure for applying an electric heating pad.

The electric heating pad is a means of applying dry heat. The temperature remains constant because of the thermostatic control. This control makes the treatment more effective and requires less time than the hot water bag. However, it increases the danger of burning the patient. There are two kinds of electric heating pads. One is made of cloth and contains metal wires; the other is made of plastic with inner tubing which is filled with water, figure 50-1. Both can be regulated with a gauge to provide a constant temperature. Pads which are "dry" and have metal wires inside cannot be used with moist dressings (unless the dressing is covered with plastic material). Pins should not be used. If the pin or the moisture contacts a wire in the pad, the patient could receive an electric shock.

In the water-filled (aquamatic) pad, an attached electric control unit heats the water. Because heated water circulates through it, a pin hole would result in a leak and burn the patient.

PREVENTING BURNS

Burns may occur for a number of reasons. Damage from misuse or a defect in the pad may cause it to become overheated.

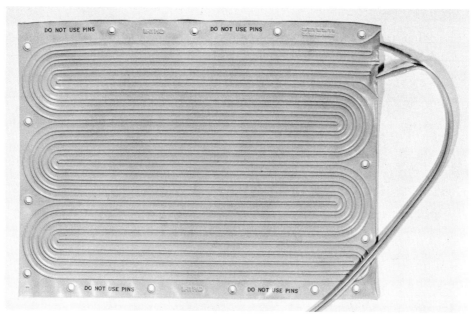

Fig. 50-1 Warm water circulates through this type of electric pad.

Burns also happen whenever anyone increases the heat above a safe level; sometimes patients or visitors may do this without realizing the dangers. The body adjusts to the heat and the patient loses an accurate sense of the temperature. This loss of feeling may also occur if a patient lies against a pad too long. The constant temperature even at a safe level may cause burns if the treatment is not correctly timed.

All electric pads must be covered with a towel or cloth cover. No pad should ever be placed directly on the patient's skin without a cover. Also, the patient should not lie on the pad. Treatments must be timed and the patient's skin checked at least every fifteen minutes. As with other applications of heat, a doctor's order is always required. The doctor's order usually indicates how long the pad should be applied.

PROCEDURE

1. Assemble equipment:

   Electric heating pad
   Towel or cloth cover

   Make certain hands are dry. Check cord, socket and switch for any exposed electric wires.

VOCABULARY

- Define the following words:

  aquamatic
  thermostatic control

SUGGESTED ACTIVITIES

- Make arrangements to visit a local hospital or health supply store. Under supervision, observe and practice regulating the thermostatic control gauge on an electric heating pad.

- With the aid of the instructor, observe how a water-filled electric pad is operated and controlled.

2. Greet patient and explain procedure. Bring heating pad to unit and plug it in.

   Caution the patient against lying on the pad.

3. Turn switch to "high" to test that it is heating.

4. Turn down to proper temperature.

5. Apply cloth cover or towel.

   Be sure to cover all surfaces of the pad.

6. Place on area as ordered.

   Never use pins. This may cause a short circuit or a leak.

7. Check patient's condition at least every 15 minutes to prevent burns.

   Remove the pad at once if it becomes too hot for the patient.

8. After completing the treatment, remove the pad, and wipe it clean. Discard the cover in the laundry chute.

9. Record the time and length of the treatment. Record and report any unusual observations.

REVIEW

A. Select the *best* answer.

1. One advantage electric heating pads have over the hot water bag is the

    a. pad can be pinned to the bedsheet
    b. temperature can be kept constant
    c. pad can not burn the patient
    d. pad has a simpler design

2. Pins must not be used with electric heating pads because they can

    a. cause a leak   c. damage the pad function
    b. cause an electric shock   d. all of the above

3. Burns may occur when a patient

    a. increases the temperature of the pad
    b. lies directly against the pad
    c. uses the treatment longer than prescribed
    d. all of the above

4. The thermostatic control of any electric heating pad

    a. protects the patient from becoming burned
    b. is intended for the patient's use
    c. regulates the pad temperature
    d. is the body's way of adjusting to heat

5. Moist dressings must not come in direct contact with the

    a. hot water electric pad   c. skin of the patient
    b. pad with metal heating wires   d. control gauge

B. Briefly answer the following questions.

1. Describe the correct procedure for applying an electric heating pad.

2. List three safety precautions to follow whenever an electric heating pad is used.

unit 51 the heat cradle

OBJECTIVES

After studying this unit, the student will be able to:

- Give four examples of devices which transfer heat through space.

- State reasons for using a heat cradle.

- Describe how to position the heat cradle correctly and safely.

- Explain what affects the amount of heat applied to an area.

Light bulbs may be used to transfer heat through space (radiation). Examples of heat by radiation are bed lamps, heating lamps, infrared lamps, and ultraviolet lamps. The heat cradle is used to apply dry heat which is transferred by way of light bulbs. It consists of a semi-circular bed frame with one or more light bulbs attached to it, figure 51-1. The bulbs are encased in wire; this precaution, and keeping a distance of about 2 feet between the bulbs and the patient, protects him from contact with the bulbs. Usually 25-watt light bulbs are used in heat cradles. However, the amount of heat applied is affected by: (1) the size, number, and kind of light bulbs and (2) the distance between the source of light and the exposed area being treated. For example, from 40- to 60-watt bulbs might be ordered if the distance is over 60 cm (2 feet).

The heat cradle is used only by order of the doctor. The treatment promotes wound healing and stimulates circulation in a localized area. It may also provide general warmth for the patient. Because of its shape, a heat

Fig. 51-1 Heat cradle

cradle can be easily applied over casts. Some plaster casts are heavy and thick; the heat cradle helps to dry them.

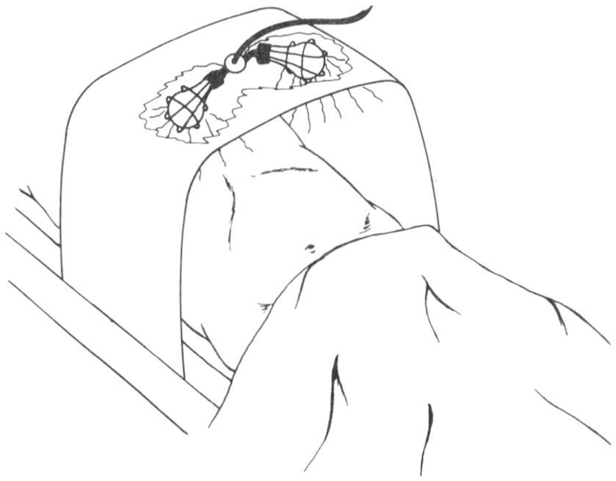

Equipment using infrared and ultraviolet light is used mainly for wound healing. Because of the potency of these light rays and the danger involved, these treatments are only administered by persons who have had special training in their use.

VOCABULARY

- Define the following words:

infrared
ultraviolet

physiotherapist
radiation

SUGGESTED ACTIVITIES

- Obtain a bed cradle and an appropriate light fixture. Set up the heat cradle and position it correctly over a bed.
- Discuss with the instructor how covering a heat cradle would affect the amount of heat received by the patient.

REVIEW

Briefly answer the following questions.

1. What are four examples of heat by radiation?

2. Name two ways the patient is protected from contact with the bulb.

3. Name four uses of the heat cradle.

4. What is meant by the term, *radiation*?

5. What factors affect the amount of heat applied to an area?

unit 52 the hot soak

OBJECTIVES

After studying this unit, the student will be able to:

- List reasons why a hot soak might be ordered.
- Describe the procedure for giving a hot soak.

The hot soak is used to provide local application of moist heat. Usually this application is used to soak an arm, hand, or foot. The limb is completely immersed in the water. A tub or deep basin is often used for the foot and a long, narrow tub is used for the arm. A fitted cover or towel placed over the basins helps retain the heat.

Care must be taken to see that the patient's legs and feet are kept warm and that the proper temperature of the water is maintained. If the patient is able to sit in a chair for the foot soak, the floor may be protected with newspapers or towels. The foot tub can be placed on a footstool which has been covered with paper or a towel.

USES OF THE HOT SOAK

The hot soak may be ordered to stimulate circulation, or encourage formation of pus. It also relaxes tense muscles, relieves pain, and reduces inflammation. The hot soak is also a way to apply medication. Wounds (such as leg burns) are often cleaned using a soak; the water loosens and cleans tissues without applying pressure to the area. Whenever the wound is an open one, a sterile tub is used for the soak.

PROCEDURE

1. Assemble supplies:

    Tub or basin
    Pitcher of warm water
    Medication or other solution if ordered
    3 bath towels
    1 blanket
    Bath thermometer

2. Screen the unit.

3. Place a chair or wheelchair near the bed.

    Lock the wheels, if a wheelchair is used.

4. Help the patient into the chair if he is allowed to be out of bed.

    Use correct body mechanics. Give the patient any necessary support.

5. Wrap the patient with a blanket. Support the back with pillows if necessary.

    Patients tolerate the procedure better if they are comfortable and warm.

6. Fill the tub half-full with water and test the temperature of the water.

    A half-full tub will not overflow when the foot is placed in it.

7. Adjust the temperature of the water so that it is between 100-110°F (38-43°C).

    Check the doctor's order to see if a specific temperature has been prescribed.

8. Place a towel on the floor under the patient's feet. If only one foot is to be soaked, place a slipper on the other foot.

227

9. Place the basin of water on the towel. Ask the patient to immerse the foot. Cover the foot and basin with a towel to retain the heat.

If the water feels hot to the patient, help the patient remove foot from the tub at once. Sensitivity to heat varies with the person.

10. Discontinue the hot soak within 15 to 20 minutes unless the order says otherwise.

Add warm water to maintain the correct temperature during the soaking period.

11. Remove the patient's foot from the tub and dry it well. Apply powder or lotion unless special medication has been ordered.

Special foot care is given at this time. (If the patient feels weak or is very tired, help him back to bed.)

12. Take the basin away and empty its contents.

13. Remove the slipper from the untreated foot and assist the patient into bed.

14. Record the time and the length of the treatment. If a wound was soaked, describe the effect of the soak.

Report any unusual skin reactions or changes in the patient's condition.

GIVING HOT SOAKS TO PATIENTS ON BEDREST

Not all patients will be permitted to receive a hot soak while sitting in a chair. Patients who are on bedrest can be given the treatment without getting out of bed. Be sure the patient is alert and strong enough to maintain the position prescribed.

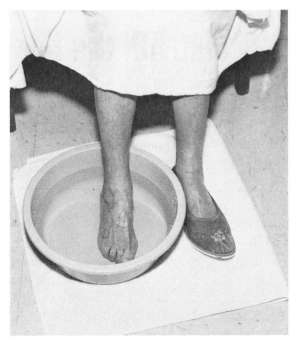

Fig. 52-1 Soaking the foot helps stimulate circulation to the part.

PROCEDURE

1. Greet patient and explain the procedure for soaking both feet.

2. Assemble the following equipment:
   Tub or basin
   Solution as ordered in container
   Large rubber or plastic sheet
   2 bath blankets
   Extra pitcher of hot water
   2 bath towels
   Bath thermometer

3. Screen the unit.

4. Have patient flex knees. Loosen the top bedclothes at the foot of the bed and fold them back, just below the patient's knees.

5. To make bed protector, place the rubber sheet across foot of bed. Place bath blanket folded in half, top half fanfolded toward foot of bed, over rubber sheet. Place towel on blanket and a hot water bottle at lower edge of towel.

6. Raise the patient's feet. Draw the rubber sheet, bath blanket and a bath towel up under legs and feet of patient. Bring upper half of bath blanket over feet.

7. Fill tub half-full of water and place it lengthwise at foot of bed.

   Temperature should be 100-110°F (38-43°C) unless otherwise ordered.

8. Raising the feet with one hand, pull the tub under them. Gradually immerse the feet. Place a towel between edge of tub and the legs.

9. Draw the bath blanket up over the knees and fold it over from each side. Bring top covers over the foot of bed to retain the heat in the tub.

10. Add warm water as necessary to maintain desired temperature.

11. Discontinue the treatment within 15 or 20 minutes.

12. Remove the patient's feet from the tub; dry them well.

13. Move the tub to a table or chair.

14. Dry the feet thoroughly. Apply powder or lotion.

15. Remove the bath blanket, rubber sheet, and towel.

16. Replace top covers. Empty tub of its contents and take care of the equipment according to hospital policy.

17. Record the time and duration of the treatment. Note any unusual observations.

VOCABULARY

- Define the following words:

  immerse   duration   tolerate

SUGGESTED ACTIVITY

- Obtain the necessary equipment and practice giving another student a hot soak.

REVIEW

Briefly answer the following questions.

1. Name four purposes of the hot soak.

2. When is it necessary to use a sterile tub for the hot soak?

3. What precautions are taken to avoid chilling the patient who is out of bed for the foot soak?

4. What is the temperature of water used in a hot soak? State degrees in both Celsius and Fahrenheit.

5. Why is the tub or basin covered with a towel while the patient is soaking in it?

unit 53 wet dressings

OBJECTIVES

After studying this unit, the student will be able to:

- Describe the method used for applying wet compresses.
- Explain the procedure for applying wet packs.

Wet dressings include wet packs and compresses. They provide a method for applying moist heat or moist cold. Wet dressings penetrate the body tissues more deeply than dry applications of heat or cold. Dressings are applied directly to the skin. Therefore, whenever the skin is broken or an open wound is being treated, the dressings must be sterile. Dressings are often used to apply medications through the skin.

APPLYING A COMPRESS

A compress is a dressing which is usually small and made of gauze; it is applied for only minutes at a time. The compress is moistened every 2 minutes to maintain the correct temperature. Because the compress is small, it changes temperature quickly. The treatment requires no more than 10 to 15 minutes.

PROCEDURE

1. Assemble equipment:

    Basin of solution
    Bath thermometer
    Gauze compresses

    Test the solution with a bath thermometer. Opinions vary as to the correct temperature for a compress. Check the doctor's order.

2. Place compresses in solution.

3. Wring them out thoroughly.

    Avoid dripping solution.

4. Apply to area as ordered.

    Compresses should extend 5 cm (2 inches) beyond area to be treated.

5. Check the patient's skin between each application.

    Extremes of heat or cold injure the patient's skin.

6. Return compresses to solution every 2 minutes and repeat preceding steps 3 and 4.

    Maintain the solution at proper temperature. Check the solution with a bath thermometer.

7. At the end of treatment, dry skin and make patient comfortable.

8. Clean and replace equipment.

9. Record the time and duration of the treatment. Also note the patient's response to the treatment.

APPLYING A LARGE DRESSING

Large wet dressings are usually made of flannel cloth or of layered cotton. However, a soft bath towel is also commonly used. These dressings are useful in covering large body areas. They are often left in place for hours at a time.

PROCEDURE

1. Assemble the equipment:

    Asepto syringe
    Basin

Bath thermometer
Bed protector
Binder or towel
Dressings
Pins or bandage

2. Greet patient and explain the procedure.

3. Bring equipment to bedside. Screen the unit.

4. Drape around the area to be treated.

   Avoid exposing or chilling the patient.

5. Protect bed and patient's clothing with a bed protector.

6. Moisten the dressing in the basin of water and squeeze out the excess.

   Water temperature for hot dressings is about 105-115°F (41-46°C).

   Cold dressings require water which is 50-80°F (10-27°C).

7. Apply the dressing so that it extends 5 cm (2 inches) beyond the area being treated.

8. Cover the dressings with a towel or cloth binder. Pin it in place.

   For treatment to be effective, the dressing must be in contact with the skin.

9. Maintain the correct temperature of the dressing.

   A hot water bag placed against the dressing keeps it warm longer.

   An ice bag will help maintain the temperature of a cold dressing.

10. Check the patient's skin under the dressing about five minutes after applying it. Remove if necessary.

    Be sure the hot dressing does not burn the patient. A dressing which is too cold will cause the skin to become numb and white.

11. Add water to the dressing to maintain the correct temperature.

    Check the patient's skin each time fresh water is applied.

12. Remove the dressing when the doctor's order indicates.

    Hot or cold dressings must be changed at least every 24 hours.

13. Clean and replace equipment according to hospital policy.

14. Record the time and duration of the dressing application.

    Report any unusual observations.

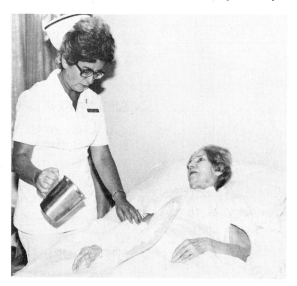

Fig. 53-1 Towel dressing being moistened with water or solution which has been tested for the correct temperature.

VOCABULARY

- Define the following words:

  compress   centimeter

SUGGESTED ACTIVITY

- Ask another student to role play as a patient. Apply a hot compress to the patient's arm. Follow the steps described in this unit.

REVIEW

Select the *best* answer.

1. Moist dressings are kept cool after being applied to the arm by

   a. placing an ice bag against the dressing
   b. soaking the dressed arm in a basin of solution
   c. adding additional dressings
   d. keeping ice inside the dressing

2. Compresses and dressings must be sterile if they are

   a. applied directly to unbroken skin
   b. applied to an open wound
   c. applied by the doctor
   d. used as wet packs

3. Application of compresses differ from wet packs because they are

   a. sterile and made of gauze
   b. wound tightly around the area to be treated
   c. left on the skin for a longer time
   d. smaller and are applied for a shorter time

4. Water temperature for hot dressings is about

   a. 10-27°C   c. 41-46°C
   b. 50-80°F   d. 98-98.6°F

5. Applying a cloth binder to the hot dressing

   a. keeps the dressing in contact with the skin
   b. keeps the dressing in place for a few days
   c. prevents dressing moisture from escaping
   d. prevents the hot water bottle from overheating the dressing

6. The usual length of time a compress is left on before resoaking it in solution is

   a. two minutes   c. ten minutes
   b. five minutes   d. fifteen minutes

unit 54 the sitz bath

OBJECTIVES

After studying this unit, the student will be able to:

- Give the reasons why a sitz bath may be ordered.
- Explain the procedure for giving a sitz bath.

A sitz bath is a method of providing moist heat to the pelvic area. It is often used to relieve perineal or rectal inflammation. Pain in the pelvic region or the lower back muscles may be reduced by this treatment. In some cases a sitz bath can relieve urine retention. Sitz baths are given only when prescribed by a doctor.

PROCEDURE

1. Assemble equipment and take to bathroom:

    Bath thermometer
    Bath towel
    Clean gown
    Face towel
    Safety pin

2. Check temperature of bathroom or shower area.

    Be sure room temperature is comfortable. Avoid chilling the patient.

3. Fill tub half-full.

    The water level should extend only to the lower abdomen.

4. Check water temperature with a bath thermometer.

    Start with 110°F (43°C). Raise to 115°F (46°C) gradually if the patient can tolerate it.

5. Return to patient's room. Greet patient and explain procedure.

6. Assist patient into a robe and slippers. Take the patient to the bathroom or shower area.

7. Help patient to remove the robe. Assist the patient into the tub.

    Leave the slippers on the patient to help avoid chilling.

8. Remove the hospital gown and cover the patient's shoulders with a bath blanket. Hold it in place with a safety pin.

    Some patients prefer to keep a hospital gown on. If so, roll it up above the waist. Provide the patient with a towel to wrap around the waist.

9. Place a cool compress on patient's forehead to reduce the possibility of headache.

10. Observe the patient closely for signs of fatigue or faintness.

    Because blood circulation is increased in the pelvic area, less blood is supplied to the head and feet. Assist the patient back to bed if either faintness or fatigue occurs.

11. Increase the temperature of the water if the patient can tolerate it. Carefully and slowly add water. The water being added should not exceed 115°F (46°C).

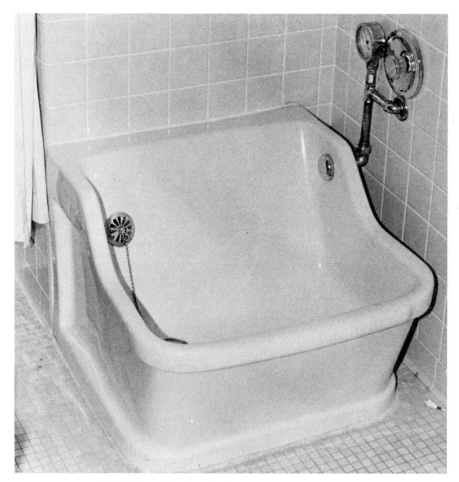

(A) A fixed sitz bath is located in the shower area.

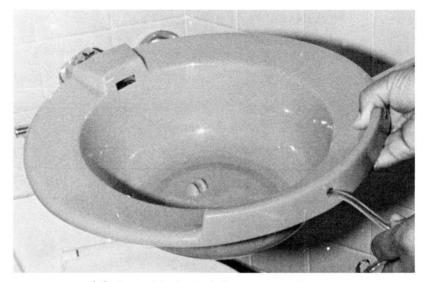

(B) A portable sitz bath fits over the toilet seat.

Fig. 54-1 Sitz baths provide moist heat which penetrates the pelvic area.

Allow some water to run out of tub. **CAUTION: Protect the patient from the added hot running water by placing your hand between the running water and the patient. Do not pour near the body.**

12. Help the patient out of the tub after 10 to 20 minutes.

    Support the patient securely. Weakness or faintness may occur with the change from a sitting to a standing position.

13. Help the patient to dry and dress himself in a clean gown and robe.

14. Use a wheelchair to help the weak patient back to the room. Check the pulse and respirations again before helping the patient into bed.

    Request the help of another team member if needed.

15. Clean the tub and other equipment used.

16. Record the time and length of the bath. Report any unusual patient reactions.

VOCABULARY

- Define the following words:

  retention   fatigue   stationary

SUGGESTED ACTIVITY

- Obtain permission to visit a local health facility. Observe a stationary sitz bath. Note where it is located to determine the privacy, room temperature and presence of drafts around the sitz bath.

REVIEW

Briefly answer the following questions.

1. List three reasons why a sitz bath might be ordered for a patient.

2. What is the usual length of time for a sitz bath?

3. What is the usual temperature range of the water used in a sitz bath?

4. Name two symptoms that indicate the sitz bath should be discontinued and the patient helped back to bed?

5. What can be done to prevent a patient from getting a headache during a sitz bath?

SELF-EVALUATION IX

A. Select the *best* answer.

1. The maximum temperature for a sitz bath should be

   a. 150°F (66°C)
   b. 105°F (41°C)
   c. 115°F (46°C)
   d. 98.6°F (37°C)

2. An example of moist heat is the

   a. electric heating pad
   b. infrared lamp
   c. hot compress
   d. hot water bottle

3. To make an ice bag lighter,

   a. remove the cover
   b. fill half of bag with ice
   c. remove the lid
   d. use half water and half ice

4. Moist heat may be applied to the rectal area by

   a. taking a sitz bath
   b. using a hot water bottle
   c. sitting on a hot dressing
   d. sitting on an electric heating pad

5. Ecchymosis may be prevented by

   a. application of ointment
   b. hot applications
   c. cold applications
   d. application of alcohol

6. Moist treatments are often preferred to dry treatments because they

   a. promote wound healing faster
   b. are less dangerous
   c. gradually become hotter
   d. penetrate the body better

7. A heat cradle uses light bulbs which are usually

   a. 100 watts
   b. 50 watts
   c. 25 watts
   d. 15 watts

8. Electric heating pads are not applied directly to moist dressings because of possible

   a. electric shock
   b. damage to the wound
   c. added weight to the wound
   d. all of the above

9. The sitz bath should be discontinued if the patient complains of

   a. faintness and fatigue
   b. chilliness and fatigue
   c. friction and vasodilation
   d. ecchymosis and fatigue

10. Heat causes blood vessels to

    a. lengthen
    b. thicken
    c. dilate
    d. constrict

11. Hot soaks may be prescribed to

    a. encourage wound drainage   c. relieve pain
    b. administer medicated solution   d. all of the above

12. An ultraviolet lamp is used primarily to

    a. aid in wound healing
    b. provide extra light
    c. provide intense heat to a large skin area
    d. dry the skin

13. Before applying a hot water bag, the air must be expelled to

    a. retain heat in the bag
    b. allow the bag to conform to the body
    c. prevent vasoconstriction
    d. prevent edema of the tissues

14. Local edema may result from

    a. prolonged cold applications   c. excessive heat to the part
    b. moist applications   d. unsterile dressings

15. Hemorrhage and inflammation can be slowed by applying

    a. heat to the area   c. warm compresses to the area
    b. cold to the area   d. none of the above

B. Match the term in column I with the correct description in column II.

Column I	Column II
_____ 1. vasoconstriction	a. small gauze dressing
_____ 2. ecchymosis	b. bruise
_____ 3. vasodilation	c. expansion of the blood vessels
_____ 4. compress	d. simple means of applying dry heat
_____ 5. heat cradle	e. narrowing of the blood vessels
	f. heat regulating mechanism
	g. permanent skin damage
	h. dry cold application

SECTION X RESPIRATORY, EYE AND EAR TREATMENTS

unit 55 steam and mist inhalation

OBJECTIVES

After studying this unit, the student will be able to:

- State the benefits produced by steam and mist inhalation.
- List the types of patients that may require inhalation therapy.
- Name the types of inhalation equipment.
- Explain the procedure for giving a steam inhalation treatment.

Inhalation therapy clears the airways of the respiratory system. Air is carried to the lungs through the nose and mouth. The air may carry dust, smoke or pathogenic organisms into the respiratory tract. When the lining of the airway becomes inflamed or irritated, it produces secretions. These secretions often become thick and make breathing more difficult. Steam and mist inhalations loosen secretions making them easier to remove.

The mucous lining of the various areas of the respiratory tract become inflamed by irritants. Laryngitis, bronchitis and sinusitis describe inflamed areas. Inflammation may occur without infection. However, secretions if not removed, will lead to infection.

STEAM INHALATORS

Steam inhalators are usually electric and produce warm, moist air for the patient to breathe. Drugs may be added to the water used in the inhalator. Medications commonly used are tincture of benzoin and menthol. The drugs vaporize in the steam and are then inhaled. The steam and the drugs soothe irritated membranes and loosen secretions. The

heat from the steam increases circulation to the inflamed tissues.

PROCEDURE

1. Assemble equipment:
   Electric steam inhalator
   Prepared medication (if ordered)

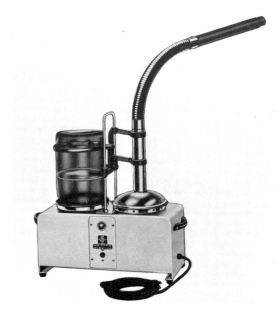

Fig. 55-1 Electric steam inhalator

2. Ask the charge nurse or the medications nurse to prepare the medication (if ordered).

   Hospital policy determines who is authorized to give medications.

3. If permitted, pour the correct amount of medication into the medicine cup of the inhalator.

   Do not put the medication in the water bottle. Check with the supervising nurse if the equipment is unfamiliar to you.

4. Fill 2/3 of the water bottle with hot water.

5. Attach the bottle to the inhalator.

   Make sure parts fit snugly to prevent leakage.

6. Bring equipment to the unit. Greet the patient and explain the procedure.

7. Place inhalator at bedside. The nozzle of the inhalator should be at least 45-60 cm (18-24 inches) away from patient. This prevents the steam from causing burns.

   If the patient is a child or a nonalert adult, cover the spout with coned paper or a paper bag. This prevents the patient from touching the nozzle end.

8. Screen the unit.

   Make sure that doors and windows are closed to maintain a heavy concentration of steam in the room.

9. Plug in the inhalator and turn it on.

10. Administer the steam for the period ordered by the doctor.

   Check setup at intervals and refill the bottle when needed. Handle carefully to avoid burns.

11. At the end of the treatment, turn the inhalator off and unplug it. Change patient's gown or bed linen if damp. Take inhalator from unit. Clean and replace parts according to hospital policy.

   If the treatment is prolonged, change the linen whenever it feels damp. Avoid chilling the patient.

12. Record the time and duration of the treatment. Record the type and amount of medication, if used.

   Report any unusual observations to the supervising nurse.

NEBULIZERS

Mistlike spray is produced by an atomizer or a nebulizer. A nebulizer produces a finer mist. Fine particles travel farther into the respiratory tract than large droplets. Antibiotics, oxygen or bronchodilators can be given through the mist. *Bronchodilators* are drugs which open the bronchi, clearing the airway into the lungs.

Various types of nebulizers exist. One type produces ultrasonic mist which is broken up into fine particles by high frequency sound waves. Another machine is used for intermittent positive pressure breathing (IPPB). This method uses pressure to force air into the alveoli of the lungs. The IPPB treatments are only given by specially trained health personnel. This precaution is necessary since this pressure can cause the lung to collapse if the IPPB treatments are given incorrectly. Fluid collection, spread of infection and leakage of air into the tissues are other complications.

VOCABULARY

- Define the following words:

alveoli	bronchodilator	menthol
antibiotics	inhalation	nebulizer
atomizer	intermittent	positive pressure
benzoin	laryngitis	tincture
bronchitis		

SUGGESTED ACTIVITY

- Obtain permission to visit the respiratory therapy department of a local hospital. Observe the different types of inhalation equipment. If possible, ask for the help of a technician and try breathing with an IPPB machine. Notice the effort required to use the machine.

REVIEW

A.   Match the item in column II with the description in column I.

Column I	Column II
_____ 1. inflamed larynx	a. nebulize
_____ 2. to produce a fine mist	b. 45-60 cm (18-24″)
_____ 3. a drug which clears the bronchi	c. 15-25 cm (6-10″)
_____ 4. equipment which uses positive pressure	d. laryngitis
_____ 5. patient's distance from steam nozzle	e. PEEP
	f. bronchodilator
	g. IPPB
	h. vasoconstrictor

B.   Briefly answer the following questions.

1.   Name two ways that steam inhalation benefits the patient.

2.   What danger exists with the steam inhalator?

3. Why are IPPB treatments only given by specially trained health personnel?

4. Why is inhalation equipment designed to produce a fine mist rather than large water droplets?

5. What danger exists with thick secretions that remain in the body?

unit 56 postural drainage

OBJECTIVES

After studying this unit, the student will be able to:

- Define postural drainage.
- Describe the way the patient is positioned for postural drainage.
- Explain the procedure for postural drainage.

Postural drainage is the use of gravity to drain secretions from the chest. Secretions which drain toward the mouth can be coughed up with greater ease. The patient lies on the back, the side or the abdomen. In all positions, the patient's head should be about 46 cm (18 inches) lower than the base of the lungs.

POSITIONING THE PATIENT IN BED

Most hospital beds can be adjusted for postural drainage. The head of the bed can be dropped to lower the patient's upper trunk. Raising the knee rest can also be done. In this position, the patient would lie bent over the raised mattress. If the mattress position cannot be changed, the bed can be used flat. The elevation is created by pillows which are piled underneath the patient's abdomen. This position is shown in figure 56-1. Another way to use the flat bed is to raise the bed and place a chair near the bedside. The patient then lies on the bed crosswise and rests both arms and the head on the chair. This position may be difficult for patients who are weak or elderly, however.

ASSISTING THE PATIENT

The positions used for postural drainage sometimes cause nausea and vomiting. Thus the procedure is not performed close to mealtime. The advised resting period is no less than one hour before a meal or two hours after. A postural drainage position cannot be

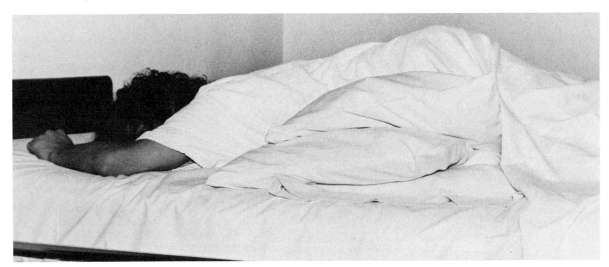

Fig. 56-1 In the postural drainage position, gravity allows secretions to drain from the chest.

maintained comfortably over twenty minutes. The nurse should stop the procedure before this time if the patient can no longer tolerate it.

In preparation for postural drainage, the use of steam or mist inhalation liquefies and loosens secretions. If the patient is not receiving these treatments, drinking fluids before postural drainage can produce a similar effect. In addition, clapping the patient's back or chest can help remove secretions. The nurse performs *clapping* by cupping both hands and making repeated taps over the back or chest surface. Clapping is done while the patient is in the head-down position.

Inhalations, high fluid intake, postural drainage and clapping all help to bring secretions toward the trachea. At this point, however, the patient must cough up the secretions and spit them from the mouth. This is called *expectorating*. Coughing deeply may be difficult for the patient. For this reason, the nurse should provide support and sincerely encourage the patient to cough deeply.

PROCEDURE

1. Assemble equipment:

   Emesis basin or sputum cup
   Tissues
   Towel

2. Greet the patient and explain the procedure.

3. Screen the patient.

   Most patients prefer privacy since postural drainage positions are awkward.

4. Lay the towel on the bed or chair where the patient's head will be.

5. Place the emesis basin or sputum cup on the towel. Put the tissues within the patient's reach.

6. Assist the patient into the postural drainage position ordered.

The position described will depend upon the patient's condition and the lobe of lung which needs draining.

7. Observe the patient's color and check the pulse.

   Do not leave the patient alone. Allow the patient to rest after a few minutes if necessary.

8. Perform the clapping technique to promote better drainage.

   Cup the hands and tap the patient's chest or back lightly. Clapping should create a vibrating motion in the upper torso.

9. After about twenty minutes, assist the patient to cough. Ask the patient to keep the head lowered.

   Provide support and encourage the patient to cough deeply.

10. Allow the patient to lie flat for rest periods. If repeated efforts to cough up sputum are not successful, end the procedure.

    Do not overtire the patient.

11. Assist the patient into a comfortable position and provide tissues.

    Do not leave the patient unprotected. A change in position may cause dizziness.

12. Provide mouthwash.

    Secretions leave a foul taste in the mouth.

13. Observe the sputum for color, amount and consistency.

    Collect and send to the lab if the doctor has requested a sputum specimen.

14. Clean the emesis basin and replace supplies.

15. Wash the hands well.

Secretions or droplets spread by coughing may contain certain pathogenic organisms.

16. Record the time and the characteristics of the sputum produced.

Describe the patient's tolerance of the procedure Note the length of time the position was maintained.

VOCABULARY

- Define the following words:

| clapping | gravity | postural |
| drainage | lobe | |

SUGGESTED ACTIVITY

- Ask another student to role play as a patient. Assist the patient into a postural drainage position. Perform clapping and ask the instructor to check your technique. Switch roles with the other student and assume the postural drainage position. Note the effort required to maintain that position.

REVIEW

Briefly answer the following questions.

1. What is the purpose of postural drainage?

2. Describe the body position used for postural drainage.

3. Why is it necessary to have the patient cough deeply after postural drainage?

4. How should the nurse plan the postural drainage around the patient's mealtime?

5. How long should the postural drainage procedure last?

unit 57 use of suction apparatus

OBJECTIVES

After studying this unit, the student will be able to:

- Explain the procedure used to suction secretions from the patient's nose and mouth.

- List patient conditions which require the use of suctioning.

Patients who cannot expectorate secretions may need the aid of a suction machine. They may be too weak to cough or blow the nose. Unconscious patients, those with facial paralysis and aged patients may need this treatment frequently. Some patients require suctioning due to the nature of the secretions. A respiratory infection may produce an excessive amount of secretions. If they are thick, they are also more difficult to remove. Secretions which collect in the throat or nasopharynx could block the patient's airway. The *nasopharynx* is the portion of the airway which lies behind the nasal cavities. Secretions also create discomfort, especially if they become dry.

PROCEDURE

1. Assemble equipment:

   > Basin of water
   > Catheter (size #14)
   > Connecting tube
   > Clean glove
   > Electric suction machine
   > Face towel

2. Greet patient and explain the procedure if the patient is unfamiliar with it. Bring equipment to the bedside.

3. Attach a catheter to the end of the suction machine tubing.

4. Plug in the machine and turn the switch on to the low suction position.

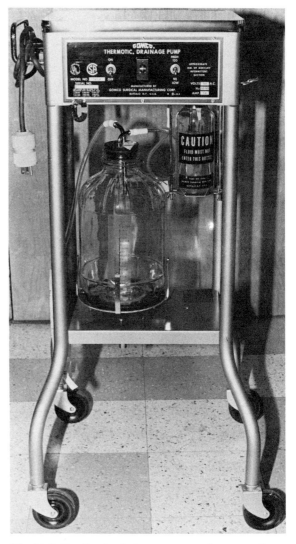

Fig. 57-1 Suctioning helps remove copious secretions.

High suction should not be used.

5. Place catheter in basin of water. Allow water to flow into the bottom of the bottle.

   This prevents secretions from adhering to the bottle and facilitates cleaning. Water also lubricates the catheter.

6. Remove all pillows except one.

   Check the doctor's orders before removing pillows. Some patients cannot breathe in a flat position.

7. Put a clean glove on the hand which will hold the catheter.

   Prevent unnecessary spread of germs.

8. To insert the catheter into the mouth, pinch the catheter closed. Use the thumb and index finger of the ungloved hand.

   This cuts off the suction until the catheter is in the correct place.

9. Allow the catheter to open and suction the secretions along each side of the tongue.

10. Pinch the catheter and withdraw it from the mouth.

    Leave in place only long enough to remove secretions.

11. Place the end of catheter in water to clear the secretions from it.

    Clear the catheter whenever it appears clogged.

12. Reinsert the catheter into the pharynx. Pinch the catheter until it is in place.

13. Suction the secretions by rotating the catheter quickly.

14. Remove the catheter within 3 to 5 seconds.

    The catheter must be removed within 3 to 5 seconds because the patient cannot breathe during suctioning.

15. Pinch tube and withdraw catheter.

16. Reinsert the catheter through the nose if secretions remain in the nasopharynx.

    Be sure to clear the catheter and then clamp it before inserting it into the nose.

17. Ease the catheter back into the pharynx. Do not force it. Rotate and suction.

18. Pinch the catheter closed and remove within 10 seconds.

19. Turn off the switch to the suction machine.

20. Detach catheter. If it is not disposable, wrap it in a face towel.

21. Record the time of the suctioning. Also record the amount and character of the secretions. Note the patient's reaction to the procedure.

    Report any unusual observations to the charge nurse.

VOCABULARY

- Define the following words:

  nasopharynx   suction

SUGGESTED ACTIVITY

- Obtain permission to visit a local hospital. Observe the suctioning equipment used there. If possible observe both the wall unit suction and the portable suction equipment in use.

REVIEW

Briefly answer the following questions.

1. How is the catheter kept clear of secretions during the suctioning procedure?

2. Name three types of patients who may require suctioning.

3. Why is the catheter pinched closed as it is inserted or withdrawn?

4. Why must the suction be withdrawn within 3-5 seconds?

5. Which area can be reached best by passing the catheter through the nose?

unit 58 administration of oxygen

OBJECTIVES

After studying this unit, the student will be able to:

- List the common causes of oxygen deficiency.
- List the common symptoms of respiratory distress.
- Explain the ways oxygen is administered.
- List the safety precautions used in the area around a patient receiving oxygen.

Oxygen is essential to life. When a deficiency of oxygen exists, the body cannot function normally. This deficiency, called *hypoxia*, can only be tolerated for a few minutes. After that time, permanent brain damage results. Understanding the causes of hypoxia helps the nurse foresee potential problems.

SYMPTOMS OF RESPIRATORY DISTRESS

The nurse must be able to recognize symptoms of hypoxia immediately. One of the first signs of hypoxia is dyspnea or difficult breathing. Anxiety usually results from dyspnea making the condition worse. The development of sweat and a rapid pulse rate often follows.

Cyanosis is a bluish discoloration of the lips and nail beds. This develops within a short time as a result of the lack of oxygen in the red blood cells in the circulatory system. When cyanosis develops, the patient's extremities become cold and clammy. If the condition progresses, unconsciousness follows and the patient enters a state of shock.

COMMON CAUSES OF OXYGEN DEFICIENCY

1. Heart damage which interferes with circulation of blood to the lungs
2. The inability of air passages to absorb enough oxygen, as with pneumonia or asthma
3. A loss of red blood cells which carry oxygen in the bloodstream, as in hemorrhage or severe anemia
4. The blocking of air passages as a result of swallowing a foreign body
5. A lack of oxygen in the atmosphere as a result of escaping gas fumes or harmful vapors
6. Drug overdosage
7. Severe electric shock

METHODS OF OXYGEN ADMINISTRATION

Normal air contains 20% oxygen. However, a 40% to 60% concentration is required to correct hypoxia. The exact concentration and method of administration are given in the doctor's order. The most common methods of administering oxygen are through the face mask, or nasal cannula. An oxygen tent is used less often because it requires a large area to be filled with a high concentration of oxygen. This makes the tent method expensive. The tent also isolates the patient from the activities and conversation of others.

Oxygen is supplied in portable tanks or piped through a wall outlet at the patient's bedside. If the tank is the source of supply, it must be opened slightly and quickly closed again before attaching it to equipment. This is called *cracking* the tank. Cracking blows out particles of dust which may have collected at the opening of the tank. This produces a loud hissing sound. Therefore, the nurse should avoid cracking the tank close to the patient. A gauge which indicates the control of oxygen flow is placed on the tank. This is called a regulator. There is a second dial on the tank which registers the supply remaining in the tank. A jar of water is al-ways attached, to humidify the oxygen before it is inhaled.

A wall unit uses a flow meter and a humidifier as does the tank. The supply of oxygen, however, does not need to be checked. The central oxygen supply provides a continuous flow whenever the equipment is attached to wall unit.

SAFETY PRECAUTIONS

Oxygen supports combustion. Although oxygen itself does not burn, materials burn rapidly in the presence of oxygen. Explosions can also occur when a high concentration of oxygen is present in the room. The condition of the equipment should be checked frequently. In some hospitals, a technician routinely checks the oxygen supply in each tank. However, the nurse should check both the oxygen supply and the condition of equipment.

USING A NASAL CANNULA

One common method of oxygen administration is through the use of the nasal cannula, figure 58-1, page 252. When using this method, most nursing care can be given without interrupting the therapy. In addition, a high concentration of oxygen can be

---

SAFETY PRECAUTIONS WHEN USING OXYGEN

1. Place warning signs outside the door and near the bed: NO SMOKING – OXYGEN IN USE.

2. Caution visitors against leaving cigarettes, lighters or matches with the patient.

3. Inspect the patient's unit routinely for hazardous materials.

4. Use cotton blankets instead of wool to eliminate static electricity.

5. Cut off the oxygen flow while any electrical equipment is in use, such as an X-ray or electrocardiograph machine.

6. If local application of heat is ordered, use a hot water bag, not an electric heating pad.

provided efficiently. When a one-third oxygen concentration is enough, the cannula is used. The flow rate required is 4-6 liters per minute.

Of all the methods used to give oxygen, the cannula restricts the patient the least. However, use of the cannula does have disadvantages. One drawback is that the cannula is irritating to nose membranes. Placing the cannula so that the prongs do not lie against the nose surface reduces irritation. The cannula is also a problem for use with irrational patients. They can remove it easily and thus do not benefit from the therapy. Patients who breathe through the mouth also should not use the cannula. Mouth breathing reduces the oxygen concentration taken in.

The cannula must be cleaned at least every 12 hours since nasal secretions will collect. Secretions irritate the patient and clog the opening of the cannula.

PROCEDURE

1. Assemble equipment:

   Flow meter
   Humidifier
   Sterile distilled water
   Connecting tube
   Nasal cannula
   Safety pin

2. Greet the patient and explain the procedure.

3. Bring the equipment to the bedside and attach the flow meter with the humidifier to the oxygen source.

4. Fill the humidifier to the proper level.

   The correct level is marked on the bottle.

5. Regulate the flow to the level ordered by the physician.

   Regulate the flow before placing the cannula in the patient's nostrils.

6. Apply the cannula placing the prongs in the nostrils.

7. Place the elastic band around the patient's head.

   This holds the cannula in place.

8. Pin the oxygen tubing to the bottom sheet.

   Secure the tubing but allow some slack for the patient's movements.

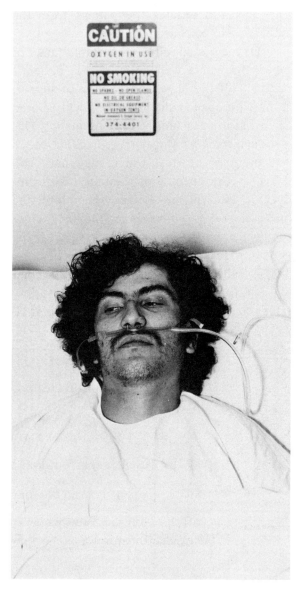

Fig. 58-1 Receiving oxygen through a nasal cannula is comfortable and unrestrictive.

9. Place the signal cord within reach of the patient.

10. Check the flow meter level before leaving. Be sure the patient is comfortable and as relaxed as possible.

Recheck the flow meter level and the patient often.

11. Record the time and the flow meter level. Note that a cannula is being used. Record the patient's reaction to the use of the cannula.

Report any unusual observations to the charge nurse.

USING AN OXYGEN MASK

Using a mask provides oxygen through both the mouth and nose. Patients who breathe through the mouth receive more benefit from this method than with the nasal cannula. The mask is also better for patients who find the nasal cannula irritating to the nose. Like the cannula, the mask provides an efficient means of giving oxygen. A flow of 6-8 liters is usually ordered. Little of the gas escapes into the room since the mask is small and fits the contour of the face. The disadvantage in using the mask is the inconvenience for the patient. Talking and eating require removal of the mask. This is bothersome and also reduces the benefit of the treatment.

Certain steps must be taken to make the mask comfortable on the patient. The elastic band helps hold the mask in place. This should be adjusted to fit the size of the patient's head. Another measure of comfort is provided by keeping the patient's face clean and dry. Moist, expired air and the humidified oxygen cause moisture to collect in the mask. As a result, the edges which press against the skin can cause irritation. The nurse should wash, dry and powder the patient's face to lessen this irritation. It may be necessary to do this about every two hours.

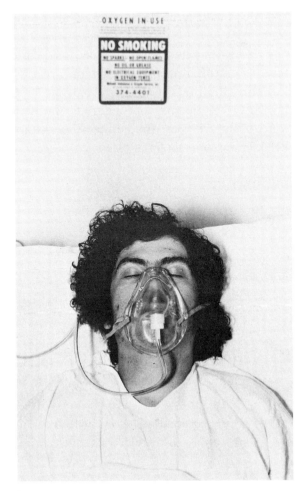

Fig. 58-2 Patients often sleep more comfortably wearing a mask.

USING THE OXYGEN TENT

An oxygen tent consists of a canopy made of clear plastic attached to a metal frame which is placed over the head of the patient's bed. An electric blower maintains the flow of oxygen into the tent. These units also control temperature, humidity, and oxygen concentration inside the tent. A flow of 8 to 10 liters produces a 50% concentration of oxygen. The tent is a less efficient means of administration than the mask or cannula.

The nurse can help keep oxygen inside the tent by not lifting the canopy too often. The tent has zippers on the sides through which the nurse can provide some types of care. Giving the patient medication or fluids can usually be done without lifting the tent.

Many patients feel isolated inside the tent. For this reason oxygen tents are used less than the other methods. Tents are used primarily for infants and children. In addition, tents are used for adults who cannot keep a mask or cannula in place.

PROCEDURE

1. Assemble equipment:

    Oxygen tent unit
    Regulator connected to oxygen
    supply

2. Place warning sign outside the door and near the bed.

3. Greet patient and explain procedure.

    Reassure the patient with the explanation. Some patients fear the use of oxygen.

4. Bring equipment to the bedside. Plug the unit into the electrical outlet.

5. Fill the humidifier with ice or water.

    This cools the tent and reduces the drying effect of the oxygen.

6. Connect the unit to the oxygen source and turn on the switch.

7. Adjust the temperature to about 68-70°F (20-21.5°C).

8. Place canopy over head of bed and tuck in securely.

    This prevents loss of oxygen or reduction of its concentration.

9. Turn on the oxygen and adjust the flow to 15 liters for 15 minutes.

    The oxygen level is high at first to bring up the concentration quickly.

10. After 15 minutes turn down the oxygen to the level ordered by the doctor.

    A 50% concentration can be attained with a flow rate of 8-10 liters.

11. Place signal cord within reach of patient and check the patient frequently.

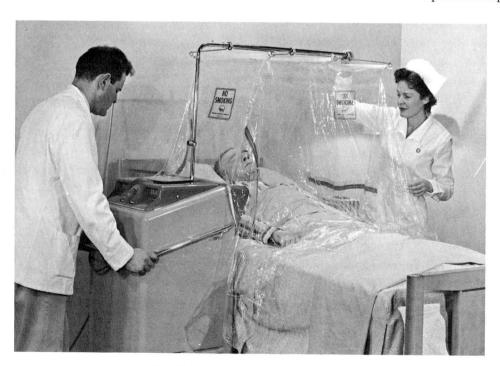

Fig. 58-3 Setting up oxygen tent unit

Change linens whenever they become damp.

12. Record the time and the flow of oxygen being used. Note the condition of the patient and the reaction to the use of the tent.

Report unusual observations or problems with the equipment to the charge nurse.

VOCABULARY

- Define the following words:

cannula	deficiency	humidifier
canopy	electrocardiograph	hypoxia
clammy	explosion	static electricity
combustion		

SUGGESTED ACTIVITIES

- Practice setting up a tent, mask and nasal cannula for the administration of oxygen. Students should evaluate each other's skill.

- Mr. Martin is a 75-year-old man with pulmonary edema who also has a heart condition. His physician has ordered the administration of oxygen by tent. In addition to being very apprehensive about his condition, Mr. Martin is afraid that he will suffocate in the oxygen tent. Hold a class discussion on the ways the nurse may prepare Mr. Martin for the administration of oxygen. How can you help to lessen his anxiety?

REVIEW

A. Select the *best* answer.

1. The oxygen source should be cut off when

   a. a hot water bottle is applied
   b. the patient takes medications
   c. electrical equipment is being used
   d. the patient wants to sleep

2. To maintain the oxygen concentration in the tent, the nurse should

   a. avoid lifting the tent unnecessarily
   b. turn up the flow rate while providing care
   c. drape a sheet over the back of the tent
   d. never use the zipper openings

3. The flow rate used to administer oxygen through a mask is

   a. 6-12 liters per minute
   b. 4-6 liters per minute
   c. 8-10 liters per minute
   d. 6-8 liters per minute

4. The advantage that the mask and cannula have over the oxygen tent is that they

   a. cause less interference with providing care
   b. deliver oxygen more efficiently
   c. restrict the patient less
   d. all of the above

5. The mask should be adjusted to fit snugly in order to

   a. form a tight seal between the mask and the patient's face
   b. maintain a high oxygen concentration for the patient to breathe
   c. lessen skin irritation
   d. trap expired air

B.   Briefly answer the following questions.

1. Name two disadvantages of the nasal cannula.

2. Why is it important to tuck in all sides of the tent canopy securely?

3. What is the usual temperature of the oxygen tent?

4. Name four common causes of oxygen deficiency.

5. Name four safety precautions the nurse should use in the area around patients receiving oxygen.

C. Define the following terms:

1. dyspnea

2. cyanosis

3. cracking

unit 59 eye treatments

OBJECTIVES

After studying this unit, the student will be able to:

- Explain the procedure for giving eye irrigations and instillations.

- State the purposes for giving eye irrigations and instillations.

- Identify ways to help prevent eye infections.

The eyes are delicate organs which require protection from inflammation and infection. The eye protects itself by forming tears. The tears wash away dust and foreign particles which come in contact with the eye. At times eye irritation is prolonged. This causes an inflammation of the *conjunctiva*, the mucous membrane of the eye. The conjunctiva may also become infected. Contaminated materials or hands may introduce germs into the eyes. The nurse should warn the patient not to rub an inflamed or infected eye. Treatments for inflammation and infection themselves may spread infection if done poorly. The eyes should not be irrigated or medicated without a doctor's order.

IRRIGATING THE EYE

Eye irrigations are given to cleanse the conjunctiva. They remove secretions and reduce inflammation, thereby soothing the eye. The irrigation is usually body temperature unless the doctor orders a warmer solution to be used. The solution ordered may contain antiseptic. However, no medication is used to cleanse the eye without a doctor's order.

In some facilities the eye irrigation is a sterile procedure. If it is not, medical asepsis should be practiced carefully. If both eyes are to be irrigated, two separate sets of equipment should be used. Solutions used on one eye should never come in contact with the other eye. The nurse should always direct the solution *away* from the *inner canthus*. This is the inner corner of the eye near the nose. Pouring toward the outer canthus allows the solution to run directly off the side of the face. The patient tilts the head so that gravity aids the flow away from the other eye.

PROCEDURE

1. Assemble equipment:
   - Emesis basin
   - Sterile cotton balls
   - Medicine dropper (for small amounts of solution)

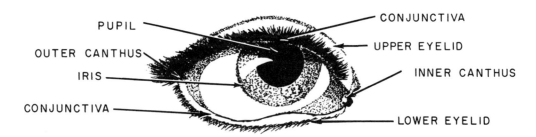

PUPIL — CONJUNCTIVA
OUTER CANTHUS — UPPER EYELID
IRIS — INNER CANTHUS
CONJUNCTIVA — LOWER EYELID

Fig. 59-1 External view of the eye

Soft rubber bulb syringe (for large amounts of solution)

Sterile medicine glass

Solution as ordered (usually normal saline)

2. Greet patient and explain procedure. Bring equipment to bedside. Screen the unit.

3. Wash the hands thoroughly.

4. Assist the patient to lie on the back.

A sitting position can be used but is more awkward for the patient and the nurse.

5. Tilt the patient's head so the eye being treated is lower than the other.

6. Place the emesis basin at the cheek, near the eye being treated.

The basin receives the runoff solution.

7. Place the thumb under the lower lid and pull gently downward.

The lid pulls away from the eyeball and exposes the conjunctiva.

8. Ask the patient to look up and hold that position for the irrigation.

The solution then touches the white of the eye instead of the more sensitive cornea.

9. Irrigate the eye using only gentle force. Do not touch the eyeball or the conjunctiva with the tip of the dropper or syringe.

Forceful cleansing or touching the eye membranes can cause injury.

10. Moisten a cotton ball and gently wipe closed eyelids once if secretions do not loosen with solution alone.

Wipe eyelids from inner to outer canthus.

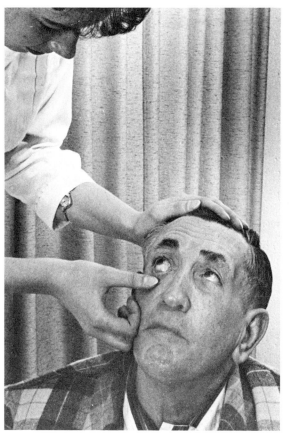

Fig. 59-2 Pulling gently downward with the thumb exposes the lower conjunctiva.

11. Repeat if necessary, using a clean cotton ball each time. Never rub back and forth.

12. Dry the eyelids with clean cotton balls.

13. To irrigate the other eye, if ordered, use a second set of supplies and solution. Wash the hands thoroughly before beginning again.

Avoid carrying infection from one eye to the other.

14. Record the time the irrigation was done. Describe the consistency and amount of secretions if present.

Report any unusual observations to the supervising nurse.

INSTILLING MEDICATION INTO THE EYE

Eye instillations are a means of applying medication into the eye. Medications are often ordered to treat infections or soothe inflammations. They also may be used to dilate or constrict the pupil. Before giving medicines, the nurse should be sure permission has been given by the hospital authorities. Some eye medications can only be given under supervision.

PROCEDURE

1. Assemble equipment:

   Large sterile cotton ball
   Ophthalmic ointment or liquid medicine
   Sterile eyedropper (for liquid medicine)
   Sterile 2″ by 2″ gauze square

2. Greet patient and explain procedure. Bring equipment to bedside. Screen the unit.

3. Clean the eyelids of the eye being treated from the inner to the outer canthus. Use a sterile cotton ball.

4. Provide the patient with a tissue to hold in case some of the solution runs down the side of the cheek.

5. Hold the dropper with the rubber bulb above the open tip at all times.

   This prevents particles in the rubber bulb from being deposited in the medication.

6. Depress the rubber bulb and draw only the needed amount of medication into the dropper.

   Excess medication must be discarded. After it is taken into the dropper it cannot be returned to the bottle.

7. Instruct the patient to look upward. Draw lower lid gently downward with sterile gauze.

   Avoid placing medication directly on the cornea.

8. Drop the medication on the lower conjunctiva without touching it, the eyelid or the eyeball.

   If the patient moves suddenly, the dropper could easily injure the eye.

9. If an ointment is to be applied, first squeeze a small amount out of the tube and discard that portion.

   This portion, being exposed at the end of the tube, is considered contaminated.

10. Apply a thin "line" of ointment along the conjunctiva of the lower eyelid, from the inner to the outer canthus. To cut off the line of the ointment, make a quick twist with the tube.

11. Ask the patient to close the eye and rotate the eyeball to spread the ointment evenly along the surfaces of both conjunctiva. Replace the cap on the tube of ointment.

    Do not touch the eyeball or the conjunctiva with the tip of the ointment tube.

12. Instruct the patient not to rub the eye.

13. Record the time. Note the medication used, the amount and the eye being treated.

    Report any unusual observations to the charge nurse.

VOCABULARY

- Define the following words:

canthus	iris	ointment
conjunctiva	irrigation	ophthalmic
instillation	normal saline	pupil

SUGGESTED ACTIVITY

- Using an outside reference source, identify the following abbreviations used in giving eye treatments:

  o.d.

  o.s.

  o.u.

REVIEW

Briefly answer the following questions.

1. Why is solution directed from the inner to the outer canthus?

2. Why must a separate set of articles be used if both eyes are to be irrigated.

3. What is the purpose of eye irrigation?

4. What solution is most commonly used to irrigate the eye?

5. Why is the patient instructed to look upward as medication is instilled in his eye?

6. Name three purposes for eye instillations.

7. Give the function of tear formation.

8. Describe how to hold an eyedropper.

9. How can the nurse position the patient so irrigating solution does not carry infection from one eye to the other?

10. How can the nurse expose the lower conjunctiva?

unit 60 ear treatments

OBJECTIVES

After studying this unit, the student will be able to:

- Explain the safety precautions used in irrigating the ear.
- Name the purposes for irrigating the ear.
- Name the purposes for instilling eardrops into the ear.
- Explain the procedure used to irrigate the ear.
- Explain the procedure used for instilling eardrops.

The area of the ear which usually requires treatments is the auditory canal. This area can become obstructed, inflamed or infected. Because it is open to the outside, foreign bodies may become lodged in the ear. Children often place beads, food or other items inside. Insects and cerumen also may become lodged in the canal. *Cerumen* is earwax which at times becomes hard and impacted.

The auditory canal may become inflamed or infected when a person has a cold or respiratory infection. Blowing the nose too hard

forces secretions into the canal or the middle ear. The *tympanic membrane* which is commonly called the eardrum, can be broken by this force. Infection or injury to the ear may result in a hearing loss.

IRRIGATING THE EAR

The ear is irrigated to cleanse the canal or apply heat. Cleansing is sometimes ordered to remove secretions or cerumen. Irrigations also help remove foreign bodies through the gentle force of the solution. Applying heat

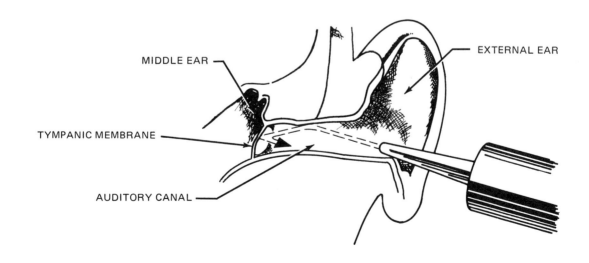

MIDDLE EAR

EXTERNAL EAR

TYMPANIC MEMBRANE

AUDITORY CANAL

Fig. 60-1 When irrigating the ear, direct the solution toward the roof of the canal.

helps relieve inflammation and congestion in the ear.

Several solutions can be used for irrigations. Those commonly ordered are sodium bicarbonate 1 or 2%, normal saline, tap water and hydrogen peroxide 10%. To use these solutions for heat applications, the nurse must check the temperature carefully. Most solutions are prepared at body temperature. Solutions which are too cold or too hot can cause pain, dizziness and nausea. These symptoms also occur if the solution is applied with too much force. Using only slight pressure avoids causing injury to the eardrum and prevents upsetting body balance.

PROCEDURE

1. Assemble equipment:

   Cotton balls and cotton pad 4″ by 4″
   Emesis basin
   Paper bag
   Protective sheet and bath towel
   Standard for irrigating can
   Sterile irrigating can, tubing and irrigating tip
   Sterile pitcher with solution 95-105°F (35-40.6°C)
   (A bulb syringe or an Asepto syringe may be used instead of the irrigating setup above)

2. Greet patient and explain procedure. Bring equipment to bedside. Screen the unit.

3. Assist the patient to sit on the side of the bed or in a chair near the bedside.

   Do not leave a weak patient unattended.

4. Drape the shoulders with a protective sheet and bath towel.

5. Have patient hold emesis basin in place.

   Just below the ear and against the neck.

6. Hang irrigating can on a pole or standard 15 cm (6 inches) above the ear.

   Never hang the can any higher. Too much pressure can injure the eardrum.

7. Attach sterile irrigating tip and expel air from tubing by allowing solution to run through.

   If air is injected into ear it causes discomfort.

8. Insert the irrigating tip into ear only about .5 cm (1/4 inch).

   Direct it toward the roof of the canal.

9. Straighten the external auditory canal so that the solution can reach all areas.

   Pull the external ear upward and backward in an adult. For a child, pull the earlobe downward and backward.

10. Irrigate the ear. Allow a space for the solution to circulate back out of the ear.

    Prevent pressure buildup in the canal.

11. When irrigation is completed, dry the external ear with cotton balls. Assist the patient to lie on the affected side to allow the solution to drain.

12. Record the time the irrigation was done. Note the type and amount of solution used. Record the patient's reaction to the procedure.

    Report any unusual observations to the charge nurse.

13. Clean and replace equipment according to hospital policy.

INSTILLING EARDROPS

Medication can be applied to the ear directly with eardrops. They may be ordered to soften cerumen, reduce inflammation or fight infection. Drops may also be ordered to kill an insect lodged in the canal.

Solution or medication used for eardrops should be warmed to body temperature. This prevents the discomfort which occurs with the use of cold drops. To soften cerumen, the doctor may order hydrogen peroxide, an oil preparation, or cerumen drops (sodium bicarbonate, glycerin and water). Drops used for an infection often contain an antibiotic. The nurse should check the doctor's order carefully before using any medication.

PROCEDURE

1. Assemble equipment:

    Basin
    Medication as ordered
    Sterile medicine dropper
    Extra medicine dropper if both ears
        require treatment
    Tissue

   Some medication is packaged with its own dropper.

2. Greet patient and explain procedure. Bring equipment to bedside. Screen the unit.

3. Assist the patient to sit on the side of the bed or in a chair. Tilt the head so the ear being treated faces upward.

4. Warm the medication in a basin of warm water.

   Warm to about body temperature.

5. Draw the medication into the dropper.

   After medication is drawn, point downward to prevent medication from entering rubber bulb.

6. Straighten external auditory canal.

   Pull the ear upward and backward for an adult, downward and backward for a child.

7. Place the tip of the dropper at the opening of the canal.

8. Drop medication into the ear.

   Insert only the number of drops indicated in the doctor's order.

9. Ask the patient to sit with the head tilted for 5-15 minutes.

   This prevents the medication from flowing back out of the ear.

10. If ordered, instill medication into the other ear. Use a clean medicine dropper if the patient has an ear infection.

11. Use a tissue to wipe away medication which drips from the ear.

12. Put the medication back in its proper place.

13. Record the time the medication was given. Record the amount and the type of medicine applied.

    Note any unusual reactions the patient has to the procedure and report them to the charge nurse.

VOCABULARY

- Define the following words:

    cerumen   sodium bicarbonate
    impacted   sweet oil

SUGGESTED ACTIVITY

- Study the internal positions of the ear, nose and throat. Discuss how congestion in the nose or throat could lead to an infection in the ear.

REVIEW

Briefly answer the following questions.

1. Why is it important to expel air from the tubing before starting the irrigation?

2. What is the proper temperature for a solution used for an ear irrigation?

3. How high should the irrigating can be hung above the ear?

4. Describe method of straightening auditory canal
   a. in the adult:

   b. in the child:

5. How should the patient tilt the head to receive eardrops?

6. How long should the eardrops remain in the ear?

7. Name three purposes for instilling eardrops?

8. Why are two separate droppers used if both ears are to be treated?

9. Name three purposes of irrigating the ear?

10. Name three solutions which may be ordered to irrigate the ear.

SELF-EVALUATION X

A. Match the term in column II with the description in column I.

Column I

_____ 1. softens cerumen
_____ 2. danger of steam burn exists
_____ 3. a highly combustible gas
_____ 4. may dilate or contract pupil
_____ 5. mucous membrane of the eye
_____ 6. nasal oxygen equipment
_____ 7. bluish discoloration
_____ 8. difficult breathing
_____ 9. repeated taps to assist drainage
_____ 10. deficiency of oxygen

Column II

a. hypoxia
b. saline solution
c. tent
d. cyanosis
e. tympanic membrane
f. conjunctiva
g. eye instillation
h. dyspnea
i. use of an inhalator
j. cannula
k. clapping
l. cerumen
m. oxygen
n. sweet oil

B. Select the *best* answer.

1. The purpose of postural drainage is to

   a. instill medications
   b. improve muscle tone
   c. drain secretions from chest cavity
   d. stimulate the patient's appetite

2. Excessive secretions in the throat and nasopharynx may cause

   a. difficulty in breathing
   b. dehydration
   c. projectile vomiting
   d. all of the above

3. The treatment prescribed for removal of cerumen is the

   a. ear irrigation
   b. eye irrigation
   c. eye instillation
   d. tracheostomy

4. Air is expelled from the tubing before irrigating the ear because the air

   a. is contaminated
   b. slows the flow of the irrigating solution
   c. causes discomfort
   d. cools the solution

5. Steam inhalation will aid in

   a. soothing irritated membranes
   b. loosening secretions
   c. administering menthol
   d. all of the above

6. Eye irrigations are given to

   a. encourage the growth of eyelashes
   b. administer antibiotics
   c. cleanse the conjunctiva
   d. produce secretions

7. The effectiveness of postural drainage is based on the principle of

   a. personal hygiene   c. leverage
   b. gravity   d. weight

8. Three to five seconds is the time limit for

   a. suctioning secretions from the nasopharynx
   b. oxygen administration
   c. an eye irrigation
   d. clapping after postural drainage

9. The heat from the steam inhalator

   a. decreases circulation to the inflamed area
   b. increases circulation to the inflamed area
   c. helps irrigate the trachea
   d. cleanses the conjunctiva

10. The area cleansed by irrigating the ear is the

   a. cerumen   c. cochlea
   b. conjunctiva   d. auditory canal

C. Briefly answer the following questions.

1. What technique is used to remove foreign bodies from the ear?

2. Why must only slight pressure be used in giving an ear irrigation?

3. Name three types of patients who may need to have secretions removed by a suction machine.

4. Name three symptoms which indicate respiratory distress.

5. Explain how heart damage leads to oxygen deficiency.

SECTION XI THERAPEUTIC PROCEDURES FOR THE EXCRETORY SYSTEM

unit 61 rectal suppositories

OBJECTIVES

After studying this unit, the student will be able to:

- Explain the method used to insert a suppository into the rectum.
- List the purposes for giving a rectal suppository.
- Explain the way a drug given in suppository form produces a systemic effect.

A rectal suppository is a means of giving medication to a patient. The drug may be required to treat the rectum or to produce a general effect in the body.

LOCAL TREATMENTS TO THE RECTUM

Treatments for the rectum may be needed to relieve pain or stimulate bowel elimination. Rectal pain commonly arises from blood vessels in the anal region which become dilated. These swollen vessels are called *hemorrhoids*. Drugs may be given to reduce the swelling and relieve the related pain. Drugs may also be given to soothe tissue irritated by diarrhea.

To stimulate removal of wastes, suppositories of glycerin or soap can be used. These, among other possible drugs, soften the stool to facilitate removal.

DRUGS PREPARED IN SUPPOSITORIES

Certain drugs intended to produce systemic effects are prepared in suppository form. *Systemic* effects are those which influence the whole body instead of one local area. Although less commonly used, the rectum is an effective route for drug absorption. Aspirin suppositories are often used with infants and children who cannot take aspirin in liquid or tablet form. Opium and belladonna are often given to adults in a suppository. These drugs are prepared with a base such as cocoa butter. The cocoa butter is molded into a cone shape that fits easily into the rectum. After insertion, the suppository melts from the heat of the body. The medication can then be absorbed into the lining of the rectum.

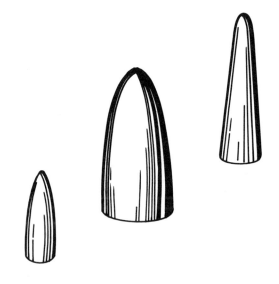

Fig. 61-1 Suppositories are cone-shaped to make insertion easier.

Blood vessels in the rectum carry the medication to other parts of the body. Therefore, the drug is distributed and produces a systemic effect.

PROCEDURE

1. Assemble equipment:

   Suppository ordered by physician
   Tissues
   Lubricant
   Finger cot or clean glove

   Be sure the medication is one you are permitted to give.

2. Greet patient and explain procedure.

3. Take equipment to bedside and screen unit.

4. Have patient turn on side with buttocks close to edge of bed near nurse.

   Assist patient if necessary.

5. Fanfold top bedcovers down to below patient's buttocks. Fold up back of gown to expose anal area.

   Avoid exposing the patient unnecessarily.

6. If the suppository is wrapped in foil, remove the foil.

7. Put on glove or finger cot.

8. Put lubricant in a tissue and roll the suppository in the tissue.

   Lubrication makes the insertion easier.

9. Insert the suppository beyond anal sphincter.

   Do not insert the suppository into the stool itself. It cannot be absorbed if it is lodged inside a mass.

10. Press the folded tissue against anus for a few minutes until the patient's urge to expel the suppository has passed.

    The patient's urge to expel the suppository will be automatic.

11. Discard the glove or finger cot.

    Sterilize a nondisposable glove if used.

12. Record the time and the medication given. Indicate the strength or dosage of the drug.

13. Determine when the effect of the drug is expected to occur. Check the patient at that time. If a stool softener was given, prepare to give the patient a bedpan.

VOCABULARY

- Define the following words:

belladonna	hemorrhoids	suppository
cocoa butter	opium	systemic
finger cot		

SUGGESTED ACTIVITY

- Using outside sources, study the common causes of hemorrhoids. Discuss the symptoms and treatments.

REVIEW

Briefly answer the following questions.

1. Give two reasons local treatments are given to the rectal tissue.

2. Identify the type of patient who would receive aspirin in suppository form.

3. Explain how a drug given in suppository form can be absorbed and produce a systemic effect.

4. What substance is used as a base in suppository medications?

5. What immediate feeling may the patient experience after the insertion of a suppository?

unit 62 the rectal tube

OBJECTIVES

After studying this unit, the student will be able to:

- Identify the purpose for inserting a rectal tube.

- Explain the procedure used to insert a rectal tube.

At times, the colon becomes inflated with gas, also called *flatus*. This causes the patient discomfort because of the increased pressure. Inserting a rectal tube allows the gas to escape. The tube also stimulates peristalsis in the colon. *Peristalsis* is the wavelike motion of the muscles in the colon. This helps move the gas to the rectum where it can be expelled. Peristalsis also can be stimulated by the drug, Prostigmin. Using the drug together with the tube helps the patient prevent straining to open the anal spincter.

PROCEDURE

1. Assemble equipment:

   Small rectal tube
   Urinal
   Paper towels
   Lubricant
   Toilet tissue
   Bedpan cover

2. Greet patient and explain procedure.

   Explain that the purpose of the procedure is to relieve discomfort.

3. Take equipment to bedside and screen unit.

4. Help the patient to turn on one side.

5. Lubricate the rectal tube.

Lubrication eases insertion of the tube.

6. Insert the tube 7.5 to 10 cm (3 to 4 inches) into the rectum.

   The tube may be marked in centimeters or inches to assist in proper insertion.

7. Place a urinal over the exposed end of the rectal tube. Loosely pack paper towels between the tube and the mouth of the urinal.

   This prevents soiling the linen if waste material should pass with the flatus.

8. Cover the patient and the urinal with a top sheet.

   Do not leave the patient exposed.

9. Leave the tube in place for twenty to thirty minutes and then remove it.

   Leaving the tube in place longer weakens peristalsis and the anal sphincter.

10. Record the results of the procedure. Indicate if the patient felt relief from pressure. Record observations of the gas, feces or fluid expelled.

    Report any unusual observations to the charge nurse.

VOCABULARY

- Define the following words:

  colon   peristalsis
  flatus   Prostigmin

SUGGESTED ACTIVITY

- Discuss with the instructor the use of connective tubing and a collecting container to substitute for a urinal in this procedure.

REVIEW

Briefly answer the following questions.

1. How far should the rectal tube be inserted?

2. In what position should the patient be placed before the rectal tube is inserted?

3. How can the linen be protected from being soiled by possible discharge?

4. How long should the rectal tube remain in place?

5. In what two ways does the rectal tube relieve flatus?

unit 63 the enema

OBJECTIVES

After studying this unit, the student will be able to:

- State the purpose of giving an enema.

- Identify the various types of enemas.

- Explain the method used to prepare and administer an enema.

Solid waste products are eliminated through the rectum in the form of feces. After the digestion of food, the nutrients are absorbed in the small intestine. The material remaining which enters the large intestine is mostly fluid and undigested food. Much of the fluid is absorbed from the large intestine, leaving semisolid matter. At times, the solid waste becomes difficult to eliminate. Irrigation of the rectum is necessary at times, but it should be performed only upon orders of the physician. Many people have a bowel movement daily while "regularity" for others may mean every two or three days. Inactivity, a low-residue diet, poor muscle tone and intestinal obstruction will affect the frequency of bowel movement.

To assist with the removal of solid waste, an enema may be prescribed. An *enema* is a means of injecting fluid into the rectum. Although it is most often ordered to help remove feces, an enema has other uses. Two basic types of enemas exist, the retention and nonretention enema.

RETENTION ENEMA

A *retention* enema is held by the patient for a specified time before it is expelled. It is ordered to help expel flatus to aid in the destruction of intestinal parasites, or to lubricate the rectum. It is also used to instill medica-

tions. Newer methods of treatment are usually used instead of the retention enema.

NONRETENTION ENEMA

A *nonretention* enema is one which is expelled by the patient immediately after it is given. The most common nonretention enema is the cleansing enema. This type is given to remove feces from the colon and rectum. A soap solution or a normal saline solution may be ordered. Soap which is too strong causes the mucous membrane which lines the lower intestinal tract to swell. Therefore if a soap solution is used, it should consist of a mild soap and a weak solution. An example of this type is 35 ml of mild liquid soap to 500 ml of warm tap water. In total, between one pint and one quart of solution should be given. This depends on the condition of the patient, and the doctor's order.

Hypertonic Solutions

Soap or saline enemas require a large amount of fluid. This prolongs the procedure and may fatigue the patient. Enemas which require less fluid volume are those using hypertonic solutions. A *hypertonic* solution is one which draws fluid out of the body tissues. In the bowel, this action increases fluid bulk. The solution also acts as a mild irritant to the mucous membrane. The increased bulk and irritation stimulate peristalsis.

Hypertonic solutions are contained in disposable enema kits. The amount of solution used is about 120 ml (4 ounces). Administration is simple and time is saved in preparing and cleaning equipment. However, the most important advantage is that the procedure is less fatiguing to the patient.

NURSING CARE

Whenever possible, the enema should be given before the morning bath or before breakfast. However, if it is given later in the day, it should be given one hour or more after a meal. Otherwise the enema may interfere with the digestion of food. An enema is tolerated better if the patient is told that it is planned. Notify the patient as soon as possible that an enema is ordered. Whenever possible, give the patient a choice within a small range of time in which to receive the enema.

An enema is never given without a doctor's order. Self-prescribed enemas at home should be discouraged. The use of enemas and laxatives are no substitute for learning good habits. Proper diet, fluid intake, exercise and relaxation together help develop regular bowel movements.

PROCEDURE

1. Assemble equipment:

    Irrigating can
    Connective tubing with metal
       stopcock
    Rectal tip, size 28 Fr., wrapped in
       tissue containing small amount
       of lubricant
    Emesis basin

    Also take to bedside:

    1 liter (about 1 qt.) of warm soap
       solution at 105°F (40.5°C) (Hy-
       pertonic solution will be smaller
       in volume)
    Toilet tissue
    Bed protector
    Towel or half sheet
    Bath blanket
    Bedpan and cover

2. Greet the patient, explain the procedure and screen the unit.

3. Place bedpan on chair protected with towel or sheet. Chair should be near foot of bed.

    Bedpan should be within nurse's reach since the patient may need it without much warning.

4. Cover the patient with a bath blanket. Fanfold the bedcovers to the foot of the bed.

    Avoid overexposure of the patient.

5. Lower the bed.

6. Assist patient to turn on the left side and flex the knees. Place a bed protector under the patient's buttocks.

    Use Sims' position unless contraindicated. Disposable enema units contain instructions for administration in knee-chest position if patient's condition permits.

7. Connect the rectal tube to the connective tubing. Hang the irrigating can on a pole or standard. Adjust the height of the can to hang 45 to 60 cm (18 to 24 inches) above the mattress.

8. Close clamp on the tubing and pour the enema solution into the can.

9. Open clamp and allow the solution to flow into bedpan until all air is expelled.

    Air injected with the solution makes the patient uncomfortable.

10. Fold the bath blanket back and expose the anus by raising the upper bottock.

11. Slowly and gently insert lubricated enema tip 5-10 cm (2-4 inches). If hemorrhoids are present, it may be necessary to use a smaller tube.

12. Release the clamp and allow the solution to flow into the rectum.

   If the patient cannot tolerate the pressure when the can is 45 cm (18 inches) above the mattress, the can may be lowered to 30 cm (12 inches).

13. When a sufficient amount of the solution has been given, clamp the tubing.

14. Remove rectal tube gently by raising upper buttock and withdrawing the tube. Wrap the tube in a paper towel or tissue and place it in an emesis basin.

15. Place patient on bedpan and raise the head of the bed if permitted.

   Assist the patient onto the bedpan and provide support if needed. Patients who have bathroom privileges, can be assisted to use the toilet. Give instructions not to flush toilet until results are observed.

16. Place toilet tissue and the signal cord within reach of the patient.

   If the patient is in the bathroom, remain within calling distance.

17. When the patient is ready remove the bedpan and observe the contents.

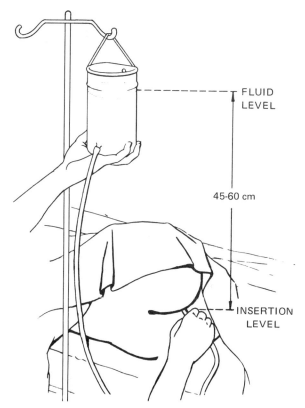

Fig. 63-1 I.V. poles adjust to the height needed for an enema.

   Note the color, consistency and the amount.

18. Give the patient the opportunity to wash his hands and face.

19. Remove the bed protector and make the patient comfortable.

20. Record time and the color and consistency of the waste material. Note if flatus was expelled. Record the type of enema given and the amount of solution used.

   Report any unusual observations to the charge nurse.

   ## VOCABULARY

   • Define the following words:

   enema
   hypertonic

   laxative
   nonretention

SUGGESTED ACTIVITIES

- Obtain a disposable enema kit. Assemble the necessary equipment and set up as you would to give an enema.

- Some physicians do not advise the continued application of cleansing enemas over an extended period of time. Using outside sources, prepare a report on why this practice may be detrimental to the patient. What other nursing measures may be taken to insure adequate evacuation?

REVIEW

Select the *best* answer.

1. The purpose in giving a retention enema is to

   a. hold the solution until it is completely absorbed
   b. help expel flatus
   c. lubricate the small intestine
   d. wash out medications

2. One reason for administering a nonretention enema is to

   a. remove feces from the colon
   b. prepare the patient for discharge from the hospital
   c. inject air into the rectum
   d. sterilize the mucous membrane of the colon

3. A solution used for a nonretention enema is

   a. hydrogen peroxide   c. strong soap solution
   b. ice water   d. mild soap solution

4. Self-prescribed enemas are

   a. given weekly   c. not advised
   b. given daily   d. administered only by a nurse

5. The nurse removes air from the enema tubing because it

   a. may cause the patient discomfort
   b. prevents a steady flow of solution
   c. contains bacteria
   d. causes the tubing to swell

6. The position used to receive an enema is

   a. Trendelenburg   c. Sims' position
   b. dorsal recumbent   d. Fowler's position

7. The rectal tip is inserted into the anus

   a. 6-8 inches   c. 1-2 inches
   b. 10-15 cm   d. 5-10 cm

8. The difference between the retention and nonretention enema is that

    a. one is expelled sooner than the other
    b. the retention enema is not expelled
    c. the retention enema does not require a doctor's order
    d. the nonretention enema cleanses the small intestine

9. A hypertonic solution

    a. usually comes in a disposable kit
    b. draws fluid out of the tissues
    c. stimulates peristalsis in the rectum
    d. all of the above

10. The best time to give an enema is

    a. after breakfast
    b. before breakfast
    c. immediately after lunch
    d. anytime which is convenient for the nurse

unit 64 enema siphonage

OBJECTIVES

After studying this unit, the student will be able to:

- State the purpose of siphoning.
- Explain the method used to set up a siphonage system.

When a patient is not able to expel an enema solution, he suffers pain and considerable discomfort. Sometimes the retention is caused by tension or embarrassment. If the patient is allowed out of bed, walking will make evacuation possible. If he is allowed bathroom privileges, he may find it easier to use the toilet than the bedpan.

If evacuation does not occur, siphonage may be necessary. The practical nurse should obtain permission of the physician or supervising nurse before performing this procedure.

Siphonage is based on the principle that fluid flows from an area of high pressure to an area of lower pressure. The retained enema creates a high pressure area in the rectum. When a rectal tube is inserted in the anus and a small amount of warm water flows through the tube, the retained solution can be drained off.

PROCEDURE

1. Assemble equipment on tray:

    Rectal tube 14-20 Fr. (Tip should be wrapped in tissue paper with lubricant.)
    Graduate
    Funnel
    Container of warm water
    Bath thermometer

    Also have at bedside:

    Bed protector
    Bath blanket
    Bath thermometer

    Bedpan and cover
    Toilet tissue

2. Greet patient and explain the procedure.

    If the patient is in discomfort, do not prolong the explanation. Simply state that the purpose of the procedure is to relieve the discomfort.

3. Set up the equipment at the bedside and screen the unit.

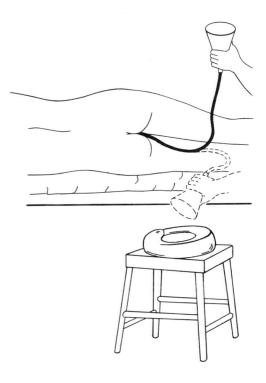

Fig. 64-1 Fluid which flows from a high to low pressure creates a siphon.

Be sure the bedpan or collecting container is on a chair or stool below mattress level.

4. Turn the patient on the side and drape as for the enema procedure.

5. Attach the tubing securely to the funnel.

6. Measure 50-100 ml (1 1/2-3 ounces) warm water into graduate.

Temperature should be 105° F (40.5°C). Test with a bath thermometer.

7. Before inserting the rectal tip, fill the funnel with warm water from the graduate. Allow a small amount of water to empty into the bedpan. Pinch tubing.

This expels air from the tubing.

8. Raise the upper buttock and insert rectal tube about 10 cm (4 inches).

9. Allow half of the water to flow slowly from the funnel through the rectal tube. Then quickly turn the funnel upside down in bedpan. Do not allow the funnel to empty completely.

Slow, continuous flow maintains siphonage.

10. Repeat step 9 until the enema solution is returned through the tube.

11. Offer the patient the bedpan. Make sure all solution has been expelled.

12. Record the time and the name of the procedure. Indicate the amount of fluid poured into the funnel. Record then the amount, color and consistency of solution drained from the rectum.

Report any unusual observations to the supervising nurse.

VOCABULARY

- Define the following words:

  funnel   physics   siphonage

SUGGESTED ACTIVITY

- Obtain the equipment used to perform a siphonage. Set it up using a covered container of water to function as the high pressure area. Practice changing the level of the funnel and the bedpan. Notice how the different pressures affect drainage.

REVIEW

Select the *best* answer.

1. Siphonage effectively drains the rectum because of

   a. gravity alone   c. a difference in pressures
   b. suction   d. centrifugal force

2. For a patient allowed out of bed, the siphonage procedure may be avoided by asking the patient to

   a. walk around   c. perform vigorous exercise
   b. vomit   d. sleep it off

3. The tubing is filled with solution before being connected to the rectal tip in order to

    a. lubricate it

    b. expel the air

    c. soften it

    d. increase the fluid volume given

4. The high pressure area during the drainage from the rectum is located in the

    a. tubing

    b. bedpan

    c. funnel

    d. rectum

5. Inability to expel enema solution could be due to

    a. tension

    b. embarrassment

    c. reduced nerve response

    d. all of the above

unit 65 colostomy irrigation

OBJECTIVES

After studying this unit, the student will be able to:

- State the purpose of a colostomy operation.
- Identify the different types of colostomies.
- Describe ways to help establish regular drainage of the colostomy.
- Explain the procedure used to irrigate a colostomy.

A *colostomy* is an operation which connects a section of the colon to an opening in the abdominal wall. This permits stool to be expelled through this opening instead of through the rectum. The opening is called a *stoma*. A colostomy is performed when a patient develops an obstruction in the lower bowel. The opening may be temporary or permanent.

TEMPORARY COLOSTOMIES

The temporary colostomy is usually one of two types. The loop colostomy and the double-barrel colostomy both result in the patient having two stomas. One stoma is called the *distal* opening since it connects to the lower intestinal tract. The *proximal* opening is located nearer to the stomach in the upper part of the intestinal tract. Stool is expelled from the proximal opening and mucus drains from the distal opening. The proximal opening draining fecal matter, is the one which is irrigated. The doctor or supervising nurse will indicate which is the proximal stoma.

PERMANENT COLOSTOMIES

A permanent colostomy usually has only one opening. It is called a single-barrel colostomy. If the opening is permanent, the patient must be taught to do the irrigation without assistance. This is vital in preparing the

patient to adjust to normal life at home. Although the task is difficult, many people adjust well to living with a colostomy. A major change in the appearance or functioning of the body greatly affects the patient. For some, the psychological impact is strong. The nurse's patience and tact are invaluable in helping the patient make this adjustment.

ESTABLISHING REGULARITY

The main task in adjusting to a colostomy is establishing regularity. Establishing regularity prevents drainage between irrigations. Three main factors determine regularity:

- diet
- emotional changes
- an irrigation schedule

No one diet is prescribed for patients with colostomies. However, foods which cause distress, diarrhea or produce gas, should be avoided. Many patients are upset after eating spicy or fried foods. Others find it necessary to avoid gas-forming foods such as cabbage, beans or carbonated drinks. Patients learn from experience which foods to avoid.

Emotional stress may cause irregularity. Rest and exercise often relieve stress that would otherwise cause problems. Patients should learn to cope with stress in a way which is least upsetting. Knowing which situations produce stress often helps the patient deal with them.

The third and most important factor is keeping a regular irrigation schedule. Irrigations are cleansing enemas given through the distal stoma. They remove gas, stool and mucus. Irrigations should be done at the same time each day. This promotes regularity which prevents drainage between irrigations. It is rare to have regularity established before the patient leaves the hospital. Dressings may have to be changed three or four times a day between irrigations. This should be done promptly since the presence of odor and the discomfort caused by the fecal drainage may hamper the patient's adjustment.

There are devices sold for performing the irrigation which are used by patients after leaving the hospital. It is wise to have the patient learn to handle this equipment before leaving the hospital. A member of the family must be taught to do the procedure if the patient is physically unable to do it. When regularity is achieved, some persons only need to irrigate every other day.

Part of doing the irrigation is caring for the skin around the stoma. The skin is irritated by contact with waste material. If it is not protected, the top layer of skin can become broken down. This breakdown is called *excoriation* of the skin. To prevent this breakdown, the patient should keep the skin around the stoma clean, dry and covered with an ointment.

PROCEDURE

1. Assemble equipment:

    Enema can with 3 feet of rubber tubing, stopcock and glass connecting tip

    I.V. pole or irrigating standard

    Small rectal tube (22 Fr.) or catheter (18-24 Fr.)

    2 emesis basins

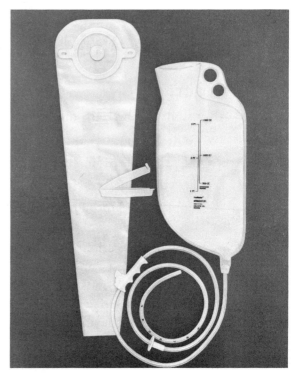

Fig. 65-1 Performing irrigations at home is simplified by use of a colostomy irrigation set.

    Bedpan

    Water soluble lubricant

    Newspaper

    Pitcher of solution at 105°F (40.5°C) temperature

    Toilet tissue

    Bed protector

    Bath blanket

    Gauze squares

    Abdominal pads

    Ointment as ordered by doctor

    Scultetus binder

    Benzine

    Mineral oil (to remove aluminum paste)

2. Greet patient and explain procedure.

3. Bring equipment to bedside and screen the unit.

4. Expose area. Place bed protector under patient. Remove the scultetus binder if it has been applied.

5. Remove soiled dressings and wrap them in a newspaper to discard.

Dressings may have to be changed between irrigations until bowel regularity is established.

6. Turn patient slightly to one side so the stoma is exposed. Support the back with a pillow.

As patient progresses, this treatment may be performed in a semi-Fowler's position. When the patient becomes ambulatory, sitting on the toilet may be the easiest position.

7. Have the patient hold an emesis basin snugly against the skin under the colostomy.

8. Place newspaper on chair for protection. Then place pail on chair.

9. Hang the irrigating can on the I.V. pole or standard 30 to 45 cm (12 to 18 inches) above the colostomy opening. Fill the can with the solution.

10. Lubricate tip of rectal tube and attach it to the tubing. Allow solution to run through and then clamp the tubing.

This expels the air and warms the tube.

11. Insert the tube 10 to 15 cm (4 to 6 inches) into the colostomy opening.

Resistance is sometimes met when introducing the irrigating tube. If it does not insert easily, wait about thirty seconds and try again. Do not force. Allowing the fluid to run as the tube is inserted provides lubrication which may help in passing it.

12. Continue irrigation until return flow is reasonably clear.

If the solution does not return after the introduction of 200 to 300 ml (6 1/2 to 10 ounces) remove the tube and wait until solution returns. If the patient complains of cramps during the treatment, discontinue the flow by pinching or removing the tube until the discomfort subsides.

13. Empty the emesis basin beneath colostomy as it becomes filled. Use a second basin to catch the irrigation solution while the other is being emptied.

The second basin can also be used to shield against spurting from the colostomy. If the rectal tube becomes clogged, remove and clean it.

14. Leave one emesis basin beneath the colostomy. Detach the tube and put it aside.

Up to 30 minutes may be required for the colon to empty. After a few months, the time is reduced.

15. Remove old ointment and adhesive tape. Clean area with soap and water.

Use benzine to remove adhesive tape and mineral oil to remove aluminum paste if used.

16. Apply ointment around the stoma immediately.

Check doctor's order sheet for ointment to be used. Aluminum paste or Vaseline gauze are commonly ordered.

17. Apply gauze squares, abdominal pads and a scultetus binder to hold them in place.

Fluff the gauze — it will conform to the contour of the abdomen and prevent drainage from escaping beneath it.

18. Give patient the opportunity to wash his hands.

20. Clean and replace equipment according to hospital policy.

21. Record the time and duration of the procedure. Note the amount of solution used and the amount of drainage returned. Note the color and consistency of the drainage.

Report any unusual observations to the supervising nurse.

VOCABULARY

• Define the following words:

colostomy	excoriation	regularity
distal	proximal	stoma

SUGGESTED ACTIVITY

• Prepare a report on the commercially made devices and equipment which the colostomy patient may use for self-care. Include cost of the products, how they should be used and their advantages or disadvantages.

REVIEW

Briefly answer the following questions.

1. What is the purpose of a colostomy operation?

2. Name three ways the colostomy patient can work to establish regularity after leaving the hospital.

3. What is a stoma?

4. Give two reasons why the nurse should be prompt in changing the dressings of a colostomy patient when they become soiled.

5. Name two actions the nurse can take when the tube cannot be inserted easily.

6. Why should ointment be applied to the stoma after irrigation?

7. If the patient has a double-barrel colostomy, which opening is irrigated?

8. How many openings does a permanent colostomy usually have?

9. What can the patient do to prevent drainage between irrigations?

10. When irrigating the colostomy, how long does it take for the solution to return from the intestine?

unit 66 catheterization of the female

OBJECTIVES

After studying this unit, the student will be able to:

- State the purposes for performing a catheterization.

- Name ways the patient can be helped to void without catheterization.

- Describe the method used to cleanse the perineal area.

- Explain the procedure for performing a catheterization.

A urinary *catheterization* is a sterile procedure used to remove urine from the bladder. This is done by placing a sterile catheter through the meatus. In the female, the meatus is situated just above the vaginal opening, between the labia minora. The *meatus* is the opening to the urethra.

Under normal conditions, the bladder is a sterile body cavity. Therefore, sterile technique is used to do a catheterization. This prevents the introduction of pathogenic organisms into the urinary tract. Unnecessary use of the procedure should be avoided since there is always danger of introducing infection. Catheterization is performed only with a doctor's order.

This procedure may be ordered to relieve the retention of urine or to obtain a clean specimen. When the purpose is to empty the bladder, the nurse may be able to help the patient void instead. Every effort should be made to encourage the patient to void. This may eliminate the need for catheterization. Retention is sometimes caused by tension or embarrassment.

1. If it is permitted by the physician, the patient may sit up in bed on the bedpan or use the bathroom.

2. If the patient's condition allows, she should be left alone to void.

3. Sometimes the sound of running water may stimulate urination.

4. Gentle massage of the abdominal wall and the exertion of slight pressure may also be effective.

5. Pouring warm water 105°F (40.5°C) over the vulva relaxes the urethral sphincter and may make voiding possible.

CLEAN URINE SPECIMEN

At times, obtaining a clean specimen of urine is necessary. A clean specimen may also be ordered as a clean catch of urine. A *clean catch* urine specimen is a specimen which should contain no bacteria from the outside of the body. Ordinary specimens may become contaminated with organisms present on the outside of the body. A clean catch specimen is needed when the urine is being examined for a specific bacteria. A catheterization delivers urine directly from the bladder to the sterile specimen container.

PROCEDURE

1. Assemble the following equipment:

   Forceps
   2 solution cups
   Large basin

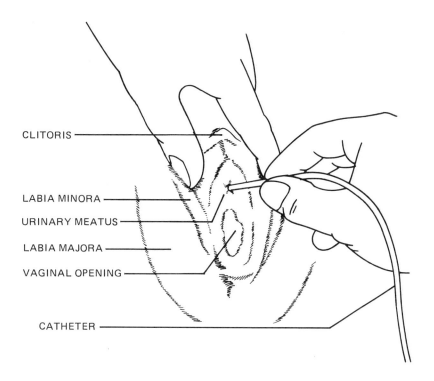

CLITORIS

LABIA MINORA
URINARY MEATUS
LABIA MAJORA
VAGINAL OPENING

CATHETER

Fig. 66-1 Separating the labia minora exposes the meatus.

Specimen bottle with lid
  (if required)
2 catheters, sizes 14 Fr. and 16 Fr.
8 cotton balls
Standing gooseneck lamp
Hemostat
Towel or treatment sheet
Medicine glass
Gauze squares
Water-soluble lubricant
Rubber gloves in wrapper
Urine collection container

2. Greet patient and explain procedure.

3. Screen the unit and bring equipment to the bedside.

4. Fanfold top bedding to foot of bed. Place bath blanket over patient and a bed protector under the patient's buttocks.

5. Position patient in dorsal elevated position. Drape for dorsal recumbent position.

6. Place light at foot of bed.

   Standing gooseneck lamp or droplight is essential.

7. Place sterile tray between patient's legs. Place emesis basin for waste at foot of bed.

8. Wash the hands thoroughly.

   Use solution approved by hospital (green soap, zephiran chloride or bichloride of mercury are frequently used).

9. Unwrap the sterile tray using sterile technique.

   Avoid contamination.

10. Pour the antiseptic solution over the cotton balls.

   First discard into emesis basin small amount of solution to cleanse edge of container. This is done to insure sterility. Solutions frequently used are green soap or zephiran chloride 1: 20,000.

11. Squeeze small amount of lubricant on cotton ball or into emesis basin.

    To cleanse opening of lubricant container.

12. Unwrap a pair of sterile gloves and put them on.

    Use the sterile glove technique.

13. Drape sterile towel or treatment sheet over perineal area.

    Avoid contaminating the gloves or the towel.

14. Grasp cotton ball with hemostat. Cleanse the labia majora. Discard cotton ball in emesis basin.

    Stroke toward anus. Discard cotton ball after one stroke. Be sure to remove all secretions. Keep hemostat away from sterile equipment.

15. Separate the labia minora and lift upward with the gloved thumb and index finger of the left hand. This exposes the meatus.

    Do not remove fingers separating labia. Cotton balls may be used to prevent fingers from slipping.

16. Cleanse area around meatus. With each cotton ball, stroke once from the clitoris to the area around the vaginal opening. The interior and exterior sides of the labia minora and the area immediately around the meatus must be cleansed thoroughly.

    Discard cotton ball after one stroke.

17. Place container in position to receive urine. If a specimen is being taken, place the sterile container next to the other.

18. Grasp catheter and lubricate tip. Place other end in collection container.

Lubrication eases passage of catheter by reducing the friction. Hold catheter 7.5-10 cm (3 to 4 inches) from tip. Nothing must touch the cleansed area.

19. Gently insert the catheter into the meatus 3.8 to 5 cm (1 1/2 to 2 inches).

    Instruct patient to relax sphincter by breathing through mouth. Do not force the catheter. Avoid inserting the portion of the catheter which the fingers have touched. Do not allow the gloved fingers to touch the patient's skin. This would contaminate the gloves and the catheter.

20. To obtain a specimen first allow a small amount of urine to pass into the general collecting container. Then direct the end of the catheter into the sterile specimen container.

    This first portion of urine is considered contaminated.

21. To relieve a patient from urinary retention, allow urine to drain into the collection container. CAUTION: Do not drain more than 1000 ml (33 ounces) of urine.

    Removing a greater amount can upset the patient's body fluid balance.

22. When the specimen is obtained or 1000 ml (33 ounces) has been drained, withdraw the catheter slightly.

23. Pinch end of catheter with right hand and remove gently.

    Pinching it prevents urine from dripping on the bed.

24. Pat the perineal area dry.

25. Take off both gloves and remove bed protector, treatment sheet and bath blanket.

26. Make the patient comfortable and replace the top bedcovers.

27. Measure the container of urine and take used equipment to the utility room.

28. Record the time and the purpose of the catheterization. Record the color, consistency and amount of urine drained. If a specimen was taken, note that too.

Report any unusual observations to the charge nurse.

29. If a specimen was taken, label it and send it to the laboratory.

VOCABULARY

• Define the following words:

bichloride of mercury	hemostat	meatus
catheterization	labia majora	vulva
clitoris	labia minora	zephiran chloride

SUGGESTED ACTIVITY

• Using a mannequin, set up for a catheterization. Perform the procedure practicing sterile technique. Ask the instructor to observe for motions which would cause contamination or increase the risk of infection.

REVIEW

Briefly answer the following questions.

1. Why is the urinary catheterization a sterile procedure?

2. Name four ways the nurse can encourage the patient to void.

3. Name two reasons for performing a urinary catheterization.

4. What is the name of the opening of the urethra through which the catheter is passed?

5. Describe the motion of the strokes used to clean around the opening where the catheter will enter.

6. How far is the catheter inserted?

7. When collecting a clean specimen, in which container is the first portion of urine directed?

8. When relieving retention, what is the maximum amount of urine which can safely be withdrawn?

9. How can the nurse reduce the friction of the catheter tip to ease its passage?

10. What kind of examination requires a clean catch specimen to be ordered?

unit 67 irrigation of the indwelling catheter

OBJECTIVES

After studying this unit, the student will be able to:

- State the reason for using an indwelling catheter.
- Identify the purpose of catheter irrigation.
- State the relationship between cystitis and the use of a catheter.
- Explain the steps used to irrigate an indwelling catheter.
- Define incontinence.

An indwelling catheter is one which is inserted into the bladder and is left in place. It may be used to rest the urinary tract during and after surgery. The catheter allows urine to drain when the urethra is obstructed. It also helps patients who are unable to control the elimination of urine. This condition, called *incontinence*, is usually temporary.

An indwelling catheter is irrigated in order to keep it unclogged. To maintain proper drainage, it is usually irrigated twice a day. Since the bladder is a sterile cavity, sterile technique must be used to irrigate the catheter. The solution or the catheter may spread infection into the bladder. Use of sterile technique helps prevent this. Even with proper insertion, however, the catheter causes irritation in the bladder. This may lead to an inflammation of the bladder called *cystitis*. Other organs in the urinary tract may also become inflamed or infected.

PROCEDURE

1. Assemble equipment:

   Sterile Asepto syringe
   Amount of solution ordered in graduated pitcher
   2 sterile emesis basins to receive irrigation returns

   2 sterile towels to be placed under and covering equipment

   Avoid contaminating equipment. Replace equipment if contaminated.

2. Greet the patient and explain the procedure. Screen the unit.

3. Fold down top bedcovers to expose catheter tubing.

   Prevent overexposure of the patient.

4. Place sterile towel on bed. Place emesis basin on towel to receive return flow.

   Make a sterile field.

5. Bring the graduate pitcher of solution and the syringe close to the working area. Remove the top bulb or plunger from the barrel.

   In this procedure, only the barrel of the syringe will be used.

6. Pinch catheter to close and disconnect end of catheter from glass or plastic connecting rod. Place the glass rod, which is still connected to the drainage tubing, onto a sterile towel.

   Pinching the catheter will prevent air from getting into the bladder. The sterile towel prevents contamination

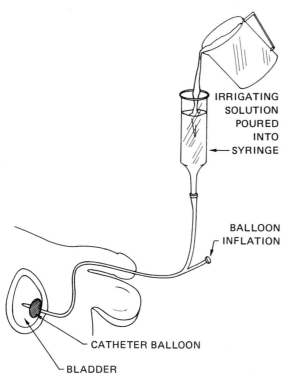

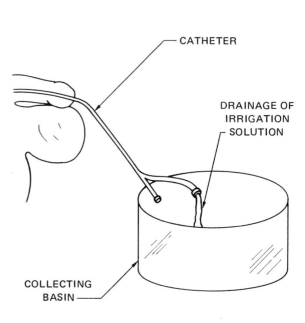

(A) Irrigation solution flows by means of gravity through the catheter.

(B) The solution is then drained into a collecting basin.

Fig. 67-1 Irrigating the Foley catheter prevents it from clogging.

of the connecting rod and the drainage tubing.

7. Connect the syringe to the catheter, keeping the catheter pinched with the other hand.

The tip of the syringe should remain sterile while being connected. Avoid contaminating the tip.

8. Pour irrigation solution from the graduate into the syringe. Release the pressure of the fingers around the catheter.

The catheter should be pinched until solution fills the syringe. This blocks the passage of air into the catheter.

9. Allow the solution to drain into the catheter. Do not permit the syringe to become empty. Pour 60-90 ml (2-3 ounces) of solution into the catheter at a time.

Solution will drain by gravity. Do not use the bulb or plunger to force fluid into the bladder.

10. If solution does not drain into the catheter, call the supervising nurse.

The catheter may be blocked or positioned incorrectly. At times, the catheter must be changed.

11. After each 60-90 ml (2-3 ounces) of solution is poured in, drain the solution from the bladder.

Avoid distention of the bladder.

12. To drain the bladder, pinch the catheter and remove the syringe.

13. Place the end of the catheter in a collecting basin to allow solution to return.

Place the collecting basin lower than the bladder to provide proper drainage.

14. Reconnect the syringe to the catheter and add more irrigation solution.

15. Drain the solution and repeat the procedure until the drainage solution is clear.

16. Reconnect catheter to the connecting rod and the drainage tubing.

    Be sure the three pieces of tubing join securely. Loose joinings allow leakage and entrance for microorganisms.

17. Replace the bedcovers and make the patient comfortable.

18. Check to see that urine is draining properly before leaving the patient.

    Remove kinks in the tubing and position the tubing level with or lower than the catheter.

19. Record the time and the amount of solution needed to clear the catheter. Note if the solution drained slowly or if no drainage occurred. Note if the urine was dark or contained blood. Also record any pain the procedure caused the patient.

    Report unusual observations to the charge nurse.

VOCABULARY

* Define the following words:

cystitis	incontinence	urethra
Foley catheter	indwelling	

SUGGESTED ACTIVITIES

* Ask the instructor to help you locate several different types of catheters. Identify the following types with a description or picture.

    a. Straight   d. Pezzer
    b. Coude   e. Malecot
    c. Whistle-tip   f. Ureteral

* Study three drainage setups. Describe them and give the advantages and disadvantages of each.

    * open system

    * closed system

    * tidal drainage

REVIEW

Briefly answer the following questions.

1. Name three situations in which an indwelling catheter is used to help the patient.

2. Why is an indwelling catheter irrigated?

3. What is incontinence?

4. Why is sterile technique used to irrigate the catheter?

5. Explain how use of the indwelling catheter can lead to cystitis.

6. How much solution is allowed to flow into the bladder at one time?

7. Why is the catheter pinched while the syringe is applied to or removed from the catheter tip?

8. If solution poured into the syringe does not drain into the catheter, what should the nurse do?

9. How long should the nurse continue to irrigate the catheter?

10. After the procedure, how does the nurse position the drainage tubing to be sure the urine drains well?

unit 68 vaginal irrigation

OBJECTIVES

After studying this unit, the student will be able to:

- State the purposes for performing a vaginal irrigation.
- Explain the steps of the procedure used to irrigate the vagina.

A vaginal irrigation or vaginal douche is the introduction of a liquid into the vagina after which the solution returns immediately. It is most often used to cleanse the vaginal area. This may be needed to prepare for surgery on the reproductive organs. The irrigation also reduces growth of bacteria and removes abnormal secretions which may collect. Applying moist heat or cold to the vagina can also be done with an irrigation.

The vagina is the area which extends from the external female genitalia to the uterus. Normal secretions form in the folds of the mucous membrane which lines the vagina. These form a protective covering over the lining. Irrigations which are ordered to cleanse the vagina remove both abnormal and normal secretions. Frequent irrigations wash away the protective covering. Therefore the nurse should perform an irrigation only with a doctor's order. Patients being discharged from the hospital should be warned against douching too often.

Solutions used for cleansing the vagina may contain antiseptics. Others contain only deodorizers or consist of plain water. Solutions ordered to reduce inflammation are usually heated up to 110°F (43°C). Solutions commonly used are:

- Plain tap water
- Normal saline solution
- Vinegar (acetic acid): 30 ml to 1 liter of water (2 tbsp to 1 qt. of water)

- Lactic acid U.S.P.: 15 ml to 1 liter of water (1 tbsp. to 1 qt. of water)
- Magnesium sulphate: 15 ml to 1 liter of water (1 tbsp. to 1 qt. of water)

PROCEDURE

1. Assemble equipment:

   Irrigating nozzle or soft rubber catheter
   Cup with cotton balls
   Emesis basin
   Irrigating can with rubber tubing and clamp (disposable packs contain these items)
   Graduate
   Bath thermometer
   I.V. pole standard
   Toilet tissue
   Paper bag
   Bed protector
   Bedpan and cover
   Gloves
   Bath blanket

   For a postoperative irrigation, use sterile equipment and sterile gloves.

2. Greet patient and explain procedure.

3. Assemble all equipment conveniently at bedside.

4. Screen the unit and offer the patient a bedpan.

   Bladder should be empty during procedure.

5. Fanfold top bedding to foot of bed. Drape patient with bath blanket.

6. Place bed protector beneath patient's buttocks.

7. Assist patient into dorsal recumbent position.

8. Apply the irrigating nozzle to the tubing without touching the tip of the nozzle.

Avoid unnecessary contamination. If the nozzle is glass, check it for cracks or chips. Use a soft catheter instead of a hard nozzle if the vagina is inflamed and sore.

9. Prepare the solution in a graduate. Warm the solution to 110°F (43.3°C) if a heat application has been ordered.

10. Close the clamp on the tubing and add the solution to the irrigating can. Obtain an I.V. standard and hang the can 37.5 cm (15 inches) above the level of the vagina.

11. Pour a small amount of disinfecting solution over the cotton balls in the cup.

12. Assist the patient to sit on the bedpan.

The bedpan is used to catch the irrigating solution.

13. Put on a pair of gloves.

Use sterile gloves for a postoperative irrigation.

14. Cleanse the perineum with the moistened cotton balls. Cleanse the labia majora first. Expose labia minora with thumb and forefinger and cleanse. Give special attention to folds. Discard the cotton balls in an emesis basin.

Use one cotton ball for each stroke. Cleanse from vulva toward anus.

15. Open the clamp and allow a small amount of solution to flow over the perineum.

This removes disinfectant from the perineum and expels air from the tubing. Do not touch the external genitalia with the nozzle.

16. Maintain flow of solution. Insert nozzle into vagina with an upward and backward movement. Insert nozzle about 7.5 cm (3 inches), slowly and gently.

17. Rotate the nozzle as the solution flows.

The solution should penetrate the folds of mucous membrane.

18. When all solution has been given, remove nozzle and clamp tubing.

Remove nozzle slowly and gently.

19. Assist the patient to sit up on the bedpan and expel any remaining solution.

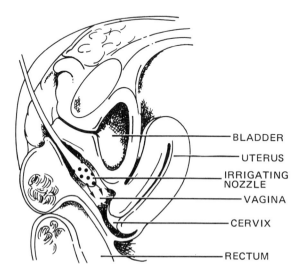

Fig. 68-1 The irrigating nozzle extends about 7.5 cm (3 inches) into the vagina.

Wait until all solution appears to have returned.

20. Dry perineum and buttocks with tissues. Discard tissue in bedpan.

21. Remove bed protector and bath blanket. Replace with top bedding.
Change linen as necessary.

22. Make the patient comfortable and remove all equipment.

23. Observe contents of bedpan.

Note character and amount of secretions removed, if any. Save unusual return and report to supervisor.

24. Record the observations and note the type, temperature, and amount of solution used.

VOCABULARY

- Define the following words:

  douche   lactic acid   magnesium sulphate

SUGGESTED ACTIVITY

- Study the common vaginal infections. Investigate the causes and symptoms of each. Determine the effectiveness of the douche as therapy.
  - Candidiasis (moniliasis)
  - Trichomonas vaginalis
  - Hemophilus vaginalis
  - Neisseria gonorrhea

REVIEW

Select the *best* answer.

1. The body position used to receive a vaginal irrigation is
   a. Sims'
   b. prone
   c. dorsal recumbent
   d. Trendelenburg

2. The temperature of a solution used for heat application is
   a. 90°F (32°C)
   b. 110°F (43°C)
   c. 120°F (49°C)
   d. 140°F (60°C)

3. The nurse uses sterile gloves to
   a. perform a postoperative irrigation
   b. avoid touching the nozzle
   c. handle the irrigation can
   d. perform all vaginal irrigations

4. A solution used for vaginal irrigations is
   a. tap water
   b. lactic acid solution
   c. acetic acid solution
   d. all of the above

5. The vaginal area extends between the
   a. cervix and the uterus
   b. uterus and the bladder
   c. external genitalia and the uterus
   d. external genitalia and the rectum

6. Irrigations remove

    a. both abnormal and normal secretions
    b. abnormal secretions only
    c. normal secretions only
    d. none of the above

7. The perineum is washed with

    a. a sanitary napkin   c. dry cotton balls
    b. a large soft cloth   d. moistened cotton balls

8. The height the irrigating can hangs above the level of the vagina is

    a. 25 cm (10 inches)   c. 50 cm (20 inches)
    b. 37.5 cm (15 inches)   d. 90 cm (36 inches)

9. When cleansing the perineum, the first area to be washed with antiseptic is the

    a. labia majora   c. anus
    b. labia minora   d. meatus

10. The irrigating nozzle should be

    a. inserted with an upward and backward motion
    b. rotated as the solution flows
    c. removed gently and slowly
    d. all of the above

SELF-EVALUATION XI

A. Match the term in column II with the description in column I.

Column I	Column II
_____ 1. inflammation of the bladder	a. vagina
_____ 2. large intestine	b. colostomy
_____ 3. passage from the external genitalia to the uterus	c. cystitis
	d. excoriation
_____ 4. surgical opening for bowel evacuation	e. labia majora
	f. colon
_____ 5. skin breakdown	g. siphonage
_____ 6. opening to the urethra	h. meatus
_____ 7. stimulates removal of wastes	i. douche
_____ 8. vaginal irrigation	j. labia majora
_____ 9. removes retained enema solution	k. suppository
	l. zephiran chloride
_____ 10. outer lip of the vagina	m. catheterization

B. Select the *best* answer.

1. After the digestion of food the nutrients are absorbed in the
   a. stomach
   b. colon
   c. large intestine
   d. small intestine

2. Catheterization is a procedure performed to
   a. prevent bedsores
   b. empty the bladder
   c. irrigate the colon
   d. empty the bowels

3. An enema is administered to
   a. relieve gastric pain
   b. relieve urinary distention
   c. establish proper fluid balance
   d. help remove feces from the rectum

4. A base used in rectal suppositories which melts at body temperature is
   a. belladonna
   b. cocoa butter
   c. opium
   d. glycerin and soap

5. The rectal tube is used to
   a. irrigate the large intestine
   b. relieve distention and flatus
   c. relieve hemorrhoids
   d. irrigate a colostomy

6. Colostomy irrigations should be performed
   a. at the same time each day
   b. twice a day
   c. every 4 hours
   d. after meals

7. The opening in the abdominal wall of a patient who has a colostomy is called a

   a. stoma   c. sphincter
   b. meatus   d. bladder

8. Catheterization is sometimes ordered by the doctor to

   a. obtain a clean specimen   c. aid digestion
   b. assist in proper regularity d. all of the above

9. Cystitis is an infection and irritation of the

   a. bloodstream   c. kidneys
   b. bladder   d. intestines

10. The indwelling catheter is usually irrigated

    a. before breakfast   c. every other day
    b. twice a day   d. after every meal

C. Briefly answer the following questions.

1. Describe two ways of inducing evacuation when patients are unable to expel an enema solution.

2. Why is catheterization a sterile procedure?

3. Name three factors which determine how a patient with a colostomy establishes regularity.

4. Explain the difference between a retention and nonretention enema.

5. Name two purposes of doing a vaginal irrigation.

D. Label the external structures of the perineum.

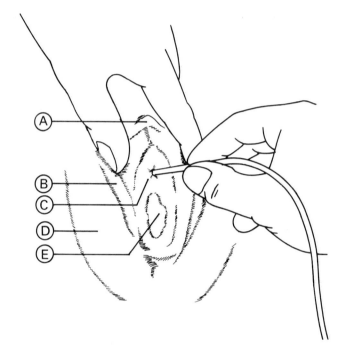

A. _____

B. _____

C. _____

D. _____

E. _____

SECTION XII CARING FOR PATIENTS WITH SPECIAL NEEDS

unit 69 care of the patient with a tracheostomy

OBJECTIVES

After studying this unit, the student will be able to:

- Describe ways to help the patient adjust to having a tracheostomy.
- Explain the steps used for suctioning the tracheostomy.
- Explain the procedure used to clean the inner cannula.

A *tracheostomy* is a surgical opening made into the trachea. The opening provides an airway when the area above the trachea is obstructed. A temporary opening, called a *tracheotomy*, is usually an emergency procedure. This is done when a patient has a foreign body lodged in the throat or has thick secretions which cannot be coughed out. Burns or injuries to the head and neck can block the airway. An overdose of drugs diminishes the cough reflex and causes an accumulation of secretions. Removal of the larynx requires that a tracheostomy be performed first. Problems which leave damage may require the patient to receive a permanent tracheostomy.

PARTS OF THE TRACHEOSTOMY TUBE

The tracheostomy tube is composed of three parts: an outer cannula, an inner cannula, and an obturator, figure 69-1. In many sets the inner cannula has a matched duplicate. These devices come in sets and the parts are not interchangeable with other sets. An extra set, which is kept sterile, should be at the bedside for emergency replacement. The doctor uses this if the outer cannula becomes dislodged.

To insert the outer cannula, the doctor uses the obturator. When the outer cannula is in place, the obturator is removed. The inner cannula then fits inside and locks into place. Cloth tapes which attach to each side of the outer cannula, tie behind the neck. These keep the outer cannula securely in place.

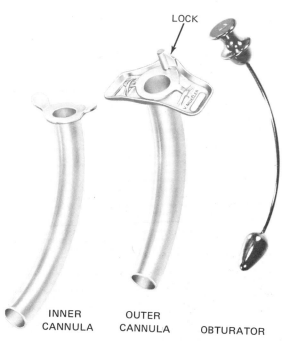

LOCK

INNER CANNULA   OUTER CANNULA   OBTURATOR

Fig. 69-1 The inner cannula fits inside the outer cannula and locks in place.

A plastic tracheostomy tube is used in some health care facilities. Some have only one cannula which is designed to stay clean longer. This type is cleaned and changed only by the doctor.

HELPING THE PATIENT ADJUST

The nurse can help relieve the patient's anxiety by showing concern. Some patients are afraid of swallowing. The nurse can assure the patient that the tracheostomy does not prevent swallowing. Secretions which collect also become a concern to the patient. Coughing is difficult for the patient but secretions can be raised by exhaling forcefully. The nurse should wipe away the secretions as soon as they are raised. This prevents the patient from inhaling them.

Speaking can be difficult since the air passage has changed. If the larynx is still in place, the patient can speak by covering the opening to the tracheostomy. The patient may prefer to use hand signals or to write out messages when speaking is difficult. Encouraging the patient to communicate in some way reduces anxiety. Patients who show readiness can learn esophageal speech. Specialists provide this teaching for patients of all ages. The nurse should help make these services available to the patient.

PROVIDING TRACHEOSTOMY CARE

When a tracheostomy incision is new, a gauze dressing is cut to fit around it and the outer cannula. The dressing absorbs moisture while the edges of the incision heal. Whenever the dressing becomes soiled, it should be changed. Otherwise secretions collect and encourage bacterial growth. Only sterile dressings should be used to replace the soiled ones.

Use of aseptic technique is important in providing tracheostomy care. Normally, the nasal passage filters, warms, and moistens the inspired air. Since the nasal passage is bypassed in the patient with a tracheostomy, the danger of infection is increased. Since the area of a tracheostomy is contaminated with each breath, maintenance of sterility is not possible. However, use of strict aseptic technique greatly reduces the risk of infection.

Secretions are difficult to remove when they become heavy and thick. One way to prevent thick secretions from forming is to increase the patient's fluid intake. Drinking large amounts of plain tap water helps dilute the secretions. Another way to help patients raise the secretions is to apply steam to the opening. Oxygen or aerosols may be administered through use of a special adaptor.

SUCTIONING THE TRACHEOSTOMY

The tracheostomy should be suctioned whenever secretions collect. This may be needed every half hour, every hour or every three to four hours. Using a separate catheter, the nose and mouth must also be suctioned. Suctioning removes secretions, prevents infection, and makes the patient more comfortable. Suctioning is usually done with the inner cannula in place. If the cannula needs cleaning it is done after suctioning.

PROCEDURE

1. Bring equipment to the bedside:

   Suction machine

   Sterile whistle tip catheter, no. 14 or no. 16, depending on the size of the inner cannula

   Y-tube (if available)

   Obturator (Although it is not used it should remain at the bedside.)

Sterile gloves

Container of sterile water

2. Greet the patient and explain the procedure.

   No matter how many times this procedure has been performed, the patient always needs reassurance. Knowing that the nurse is attentive, careful, and concerned, adds to the patient's comfort.

3. Place the patient in Fowler's or semi-Fowler's position, if permitted.

4. Put on sterile gloves.

5. Test the suction by placing the tip of the catheter in the sterile water and turning on the machine.

   A sucking sound should be heard, and water can be seen as it is drawn into the bottle of the suction machine.

6. Encourage the patient to exhale forcefully. During suctioning his neck should be hyperextended. Provide support by placing a pillow under the shoulders.

   Raising the shoulders causes the head to drop back in the hyperextended position.

7. Insert the catheter no more than 10 or 12.5 cm (4 or 5 inches) into the tracheostomy. Pinch catheter as it is being inserted to shut off the suction temporarily.

   A Y-tube is often used to connect the catheter to the suction machine. With a Y-tube, release the suction by keeping the thumb off the opening.

8. Suction gently and quickly, using a rotating motion. Do not suction for longer than 3 to 5 seconds. Do not allow the catheter to go farther into the tube while suction is applied.

The patient cannot breathe during suctioning. Rough or careless handling of the catheter causes trauma to the tissue, increases secretions, and raises the possibility of infection.

9. Release the suction and withdraw the catheter.

   Pinch the catheter or if a Y-tube is used, leave the opening free to cut off suction.

10. Flush the catheter by placing it in a container of sterile water.

11. Repeat the suctioning until the airway is clear.

    Three or four times usually clears the airway. Allow the patient to rest between suctioning intervals.

12. Use a separate suction catheter and rinsing solution if mouth and nose suctioning is needed.

    Prevent germs from the nose and mouth from being carried into the tracheostomy.

13. Flush the catheter with sterile water and turn off the suction.

14. Wrap the catheter in a clean towel or place it in disinfectant solution. Leave it at the bedside.

    In some hospitals a disposable sterile catheter is used and discarded after use.

15. Remove gloves being careful not to contaminate the hands with secretions which may be on the outside of the gloves.

16. Assist the patient into a comfortable position. Stay with the patient for a short time if the procedure has caused uneasiness.

17. Record the time, and duration of the suctioning procedure. Note the

amount, consistency and color of the secretions.

CLEANING THE INNER CANNULA

The inner cannula is cleaned to prevent secretions from drying and blocking the opening. Suctioning is done first to remove the secretions. The cannula is then withdrawn to be cleaned thoroughly. Care should be taken not to soil the outer cannula. If it becomes necessary to remove the outer cannula, the doctor performs this procedure.

PROCEDURE

1. Assemble the equipment:

    Sterile basin
    Sterile pipe cleaners or a narrow
       brush
    Sterile water
    *3 x 3 sterile gauze
    Hydrogen peroxide
    Suctioning equipment and supplies

    * Cotton-filled dressings or facial tissue must not be used since they contain lint which may be inspired.

2. Perform the suctioning procedure first if secretions in the cannula are heavy.

3. Explain the procedure to the patient.

4. Unlock the inner cannula by turning it. Hold the outer cannula to prevent dislodging it as the inner cannula is withdrawn.

5. Soak the cannula in a basin of hydrogen peroxide.

    In some hospitals a surgical detergent is used.

6. Remove secretions on the inside of the cannula with the pipe cleaners or the brush.

7. Rinse the tube in sterile water. Shake off the excess water.

    This removes the cleaning solution and the secretions.

8. If necessary, suction the outer cannula before replacing the cleaned inner cannula.

9. Replace the inner cannula and lock it in place.

10. If gauze has been placed around the outer cannula, check to see whether it is soiled. If so, replace it with sterile gauze.

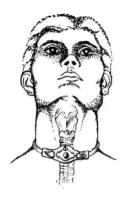

(A) Strings tied around the neck hold the outer cannula in place.

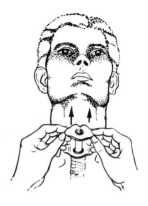

(B) The inner cannula turns and lifts out easily for cleaning.

Fig. 69-2 The nurse can remove the inner cannula but always leaves the outer cannula in place.

11. Assist the patient into a comfortable position. Place the signal cord within reach.

12. Record the time the procedure was done. Indicate that the inner cannula was removed and cleaned.

A sterile, duplicate inner cannula may be used with the next change. Cleaning the soiled cannula at the bedside is done when a sterile cannula is not available.

VOCABULARY

- Define the following words:

aerosol	lint	tracheostomy
esophageal speech	obturator	tracheotomy
incision		

SUGGESTED ACTIVITIES

- Ask the instructor to help obtain a tracheostomy set. Examine the cannulas and practice locking the inner cannula into the outer cannula.

- Obtain permission to visit a local hospital. Observe the suctioning procedure being done by a nurse. Notice the patient's response to the procedure.

REVIEW

Select the *best* answer.

1. In the care of a tracheostomy patient, if the outer cannula is to be removed, this is done by the

   a. nurse   c. doctor
   b. patient   d. inhalation therapist

2. The inner cannula of the tracheostomy apparatus is removed for cleaning and replacement

   a. whenever necessary — at least once a day
   b. every hour
   c. only by the doctor
   d. when patient leaves the hospital

3. The tracheostomy should be suctioned

   a. continuously
   b. every four hours at the most
   c. whenever secretions begin to dry
   d. before the inner cannula is removed

4. Careless handling when suctioning a patient with a tracheostomy may

   a. cause trauma to the tissue   c. raise possibility of infection
   b. increase secretions   d. all of the above

5. The suctioning catheter should be inserted

   a. 2.5 to 4 cm (1 to 1 1/2 inches)
   b. 10 to 12.5 cm (4 to 5 inches)
   c. 15 to 20 cm (6 to 8 inches)
   d. 20 to 25 cm (8 to 10 inches)

6. The suction should be applied for

   a. 3 to 5 seconds at a time   c. 2 to 3 minutes
   b. 20 to 30 seconds at a time   d. 3 to 5 minutes

7. A Y-tube is used to

   a. fit around the outer cannula   c. produce a sucking sound
   b. pinch the catheter   d. regulate the suction

8. Between brief suctioning intervals the catheter is flushed with

   a. sterile water   c. tap water
   b. hydrogen peroxide   d. surgical detergent

9. To suction the nose and mouth, use a catheter which

   a. is larger than the one used in the tracheostomy
   b. has been used for the tracheostomy earlier
   c. is separate from the one used for the tracheostomy
   d. is nondisposable

10. The three parts of a tracheostomy set are the

   a. catheter, suction machine and Y-tube
   b. center tube, plastic tube and catheter
   c. Y-tube, catheter and suction tubing
   d. inner cannula, outer cannula and obturator

unit 70 special bed equipment

OBJECTIVES

After studying this unit, the student will be able to:

- Identify the procedure for using special bed equipment.
- Explain the advantages in using the various pieces of special bed equipment.

Most special bed equipment is designed to help patients who must remain on prolonged bedrest. Some injuries or conditions limit the patient's ability to move or turn in the bed. Pain from severe burns or paralysis from spinal cord injuries may confine the patient to one position. Without a change in position, a patient can easily develop decubiti and poor general circulation. Special mattresses help relieve constant pressure over a skin area. Special beds turn or rotate the body when a patient is unable to turn.

USING MATTRESSES TO PREVENT DECUBITI

Decubiti are a hazard to any patient who must stay in bed for long periods of time. Good nursing care can often prevent decubiti from forming. Therefore, the nurse should be familiar with the special devices used to help prevent decubiti. One device is a mattress filled with water which sits inside a sturdy frame. The water acts as a cushion to relieve the pressure over bony areas. Another device commonly used is the alternating pressure mattress. This mattress is filled with pockets of air. The electric motor attached inflates only half the number of air pockets at a time. This shifts the pressure constantly from one area of the skin to another. The alternating pressure stimulates circulation through the skin.

CIRCLE® BED

The Circle® bed is used to place the patient in various vertical and horizontal positions. Patients who have spinal cord injuries and cannot turn without assistance, benefit from a bed of this type. The Circle® bed also helps patients with severe burns since it makes turning less painful.

The Circle® bed often functions as a tilt table. Patients with orthopedic conditions can benefit from using the bed or the table. Either helps the patient to increase the strength in the back and the legs gradually.

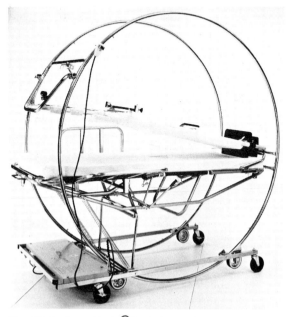

Fig. 70-1 In a Circle® bed the patient rotates easily from one position to another.

The more vertical the position, the more weight the feet bear. This helps the patient gradually assume a standing position.

THE STRYKER TURNING FRAME

The Stryker turning frame provides a simple means of turning the patient from a face up to a face down position. The frame can be adjusted to fit the patient's height. When the frame fits, it keeps the body aligned and comfortable. The Stryker frame provides the following advantages.

1. Patients can be placed on the bedpan without being lifted.

2. Patients can feed themselves or read while lying prone.

3. Patients can be transported in the frame.

4. Patients can be turned easily, thereby preventing decubiti.

PROCEDURE

1. Greet the patient and explain how the bed will be turned.

   Do not assume the patient is accustomed to the procedure.

2. Remove the top linen and prepare to turn the patient to a face down position.

3. Ask for the assistance of another health team member. One person stands at the head of the frame; the other stands at the foot.

4. Place the anterior frame over the patient.

   Be sure the frame centers over the body and supports the head.

5. Lock the anterior frame in place using the lock nut and pin at each end of the frame.

6. Fasten the frames together with canvas straps which wrap around both frames.

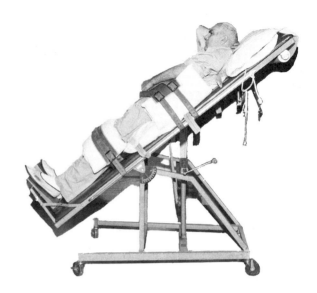

Fig. 70-2 Bearing full weight on the feet is gradual through use of the tilt table.

The straps prevent the patient from slipping from the frame.

7. Instruct the patient to grasp around the anterior frame with the arms.

   The arms should remain in place during the turning.

8. Tell the patient in which direction the turn will be made.

9. Give a signal to the other health team member and make the turn quickly.

10. Remove the straps and release the lock.

11. Lift off the posterior frame.

    The patient is now lying face down on the anterior frame.

12. Replace the bedcovers; adjust the footboard and armrests. Make the patient comfortable.

13. Record the time the patient was turned. Note any unusual reactions the patient had to the turn.

    Report unusual observations to the charge nurse.

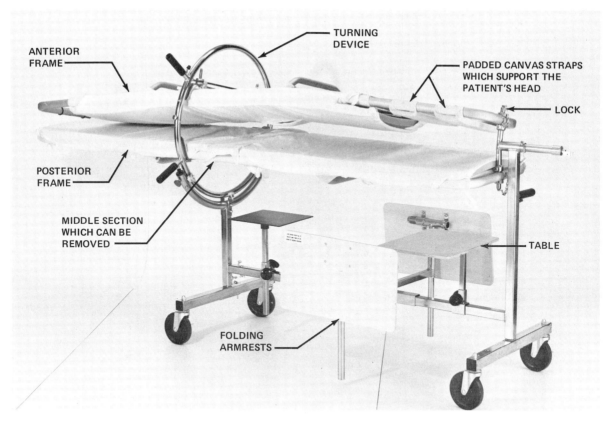

ANTERIOR FRAME

TURNING DEVICE

PADDED CANVAS STRAPS WHICH SUPPORT THE PATIENT'S HEAD

LOCK

POSTERIOR FRAME

MIDDLE SECTION WHICH CAN BE REMOVED

TABLE

FOLDING ARMRESTS

Fig. 70-3 The patient lies between the two frames which rotate.

VOCABULARY

• Define the following words:

alternating	orthopedic	tilt
anterior	rotate	vertical
horizontal		

SUGGESTED ACTIVITY

• Obtain permission to visit a local hospital and observe a Stryker frame in use. Note how the patient responds to the turn. If an empty Stryker frame is available, practice using it with a mannequin. Ask the instructor to observe your technique.

REVIEW

Briefly answer the following questions.

1. How does the alternating pressure mattress help prevent decubiti?

2. In what positions can the patient be turned in the Circle® bed?

3. Name two different parts of the Stryker frame which hold the upper and lower frames together for turning.

4. How does the Circle® bed function as a tilt table?

5. Name four advantages provided by the Stryker turning frame.

unit 71 care of the unconscious patient

OBJECTIVES

After studying this unit, the student will be able to:

- Explain two ways to give the unconscious patient nourishment.

- Explain the nursing care necessary for the unconscious patient.

- State how loss of muscle tone affects the patient's care.

The unconscious patient lacks the ability to sense or respond to stimuli. This condition may be temporary or permanent. It also may vary in depth from a stupor to coma. In a stupor, the patient may at times react to unpleasant stimuli. The patient may retract, grimace or groan. In a coma, however, a patient makes no response.

SPECIAL NEEDS OF THE UNCONSCIOUS PATIENT

The unconscious patient cannot explain needs and feelings to the nurse. For this reason, the nurse must anticipate the patient's needs. The patient's condition should be observed and recorded carefully. Injuries from poor positioning or from burns must be prevented by the nurse. This extra attention is necessary because the patient cannot respond normally to discomfort or pain.

Because the patient cannot move without help, the nurse must use the same measures taken to help patients on prolonged bedrest. Good skin care, use of special mattresses, and frequent turning helps prevent decubiti. Keeping linen free from crumbs and wrinkles reduces skin irritation. Applying lotion to the patient's skin prevents irritation caused by dryness. In addition, keeping the body in alignment helps prevent deformities.

The unconscious state suppresses the patient's sense to temperature. Even in room temperature the patient may need extra blankets. If the skin on the inner thigh is cool, the patient should be given extra bedcovers. No heat applications should be used to warm the patient. Hot water bags or heating pads could easily burn the patient.

Loss of muscle tone often causes collection of secretions and loss of control of discharges. Secretions of the eyes, nose and mouth must be cleaned away. At times, secretions of the nose and mouth are suctioned. Lubricating the nose and the lips helps prevent them from drying. The unconscious patient also may lose control over discharges of urine and stool. The nurse should keep the patient clean and dry. If the patient is unconscious for a prolonged period of time, a Foley catheter is inserted to drain the urine. When it is possible, the patient can be put on a regular urine and bowel control schedule.

NOURISHING THE PATIENT

The unconscious patient is fed intravenously or by a nasogastric tube. When feeding the patient through a nasogastric tube, the nurse should give the solution in small amounts. A common feeding schedule is 100 to 200 ml (3-6 1/2 ounces) every 2 to 3 hours. Giving small amounts prevents overloading the stomach. Care must be taken to prevent vomiting. An unconscious patient may aspirate vomited material. *Aspirated* material enters the breathing passages and may obstruct the airway.

VOCABULARY

- Define the following words:

aspirated	grimace	stimuli
coma	retract	suppress

SUGGESTED ACTIVITY

- List the equipment you would probably need to prepare the unit for the admission of an unconscious patient.

REVIEW

Briefly answer the following questions.

1. What two means can be used to provide nourishment for the unconscious patient?

2. Why is it important to keep linen smooth and free from wrinkles?

3. Of what value is a frequent change of position?

4. How can the nurse help the unconscious patient who is cold?

5. How does loss of muscle tone increase the patient's need for nursing care?

unit 72 care of the incontinent patient

OBJECTIVES

After studying this unit, the student will be able to:

- Identify at least one condition which causes incontinence.

- Explain ways to keep the incontinent patient comfortable.

- Describe ways to help the patient form regular elimination patterns.

- Identify the reason an indwelling catheter is avoided if possible.

Incontinence is the loss of control over elimination of urine and feces. It is usually temporary and has various causes. Unconsciousness and problems with the nervous system may cause a patient to be incontinent. Problems with the urinary or gastrointestinal tract may also cause this condition.

The incontinent patient should be kept clean and dry. This may require a great deal of the nurse's attention. Good care is important in preventing decubiti. It also is needed to reduce the unpleasant nature of the condition. Bed protectors should be placed under the patient at all times. The nurse should be sure the linens and the patient's gown are changed whenever damp or soiled.

An indwelling catheter is sometimes ordered to drain the patient's urine. The physician decides whether the catheter is inserted.

Because catheters can lead to infections in the bladder, many doctors try to avoid their use. The nurse can help the patient empty the bladder regularly. This is done by making a record of whenever the patient urinates. The record usually shows a pattern of the patient's elimination habits. The nurse can give the patient a urinal or bedpan whenever the pattern shows the patient is likely to need it. Regular emptying of the bladder helps reduce the problems of incontinence.

In many cases, fecal incontinence can be regulated if a pattern is formed. Use of enemas, cathartics and increased fluid intake can help regulate the bowels. When medications or enemas are given at the same time each day, they help establish a pattern. This helps prevent involuntary stools.

VOCABULARY

- Define the following words:

  cathartics   gastrointestinal   involuntary

SUGGESTED ACTIVITY

- Study the use of bladder and bowel training programs. Discuss with the instructor the procedure for establishing one with a patient in a hospital setting.

REVIEW

Select the *best* answer.

1. The incontinent patient is kept clean and dry by

   a. changing damp or soiled linens
   b. using bed protectors
   c. checking to see that the gown is not damp
   d. all of the above

2. Incontinence is defined as the loss of control over elimination of

   a. urine
   b. feces
   c. urine and feces
   d. none of the above

3. Enemas and cathartics given at the same time each day help

   a. prevent involuntary stools
   b. improve the patient's bladder training
   c. decrease the patient's stay in the hospital
   d. reduce the need for a catheter

4. The use of a urinary catheter is avoided when possible because

   a. only the supervising nurse can order it to be inserted
   b. it increases the occurrence of bladder infections
   c. cathartics eliminate the need for it
   d. it disturbs bowel movement patterns

5. A condition which often causes incontinence is

   a. pregnancy
   b. ulcers
   c. unconsciousness
   d. mental illness

unit 73 feeding the patient

OBJECTIVES

After studying this unit, the student will be able to:

- State important points to follow when feeding a patient by mouth.
- Explain the steps used to give a nasogastric tube feeding.

Patients who cannot feed themselves require the assistance of a nurse. Nourishment can be given through an I.V., a nasogastric tube or by mouth. The patient's condition determines which method is used. The doctor orders the type of nourishment and the means by which it is given. Whatever method is used, the nurse should use an unhurried manner. The patient should be as relaxed as possible when being fed. This helps the patient digest the food or nourishment. It also makes mealtime more pleasant.

FEEDING THE PATIENT BY MOUTH

Some patients are alert and able to eat a regular diet but cannot feed themselves. Some patients cannot use their arms or hands due to a stroke, burns, fractures or various other conditions. The condition may not affect the patient's appetite or the desire for a relaxing meal. The nurse should make an effort to help the patient enjoy mealtime. If the nurse sits as she feeds the patient, it will give the patient a relaxed, unhurried feeling.

PROCEDURE

1. Assemble items needed to prepare the patient for a meal:

Bedpan or urinal	Soap
Face cloth	Basin
Towel	Food tray

2. Greet and inform the patient that the food tray will arrive shortly.

3. Offer the patient the bedpan or urinal. Assist if necessary.

4. Assist the patient into a sitting position, if permitted.

   A dangling position is not used unless the patient is strong enough to remain there during the whole meal.

5. Clear the overbed table and place it near the patient.

6. Place the towels, soap and basin of warm water on the overbed table. Assist the patient to wash the hands and face.

   Allow the patient to do as much as possible without help.

7. Assist the patient into a comfortable position for eating. Support the patient with pillows if needed.

8. Bring the food tray to the bedside so the patient can see it. Check to see that the correct name and diet is labeled on the tray.

   The sight and smell of food often helps stimulate the appetite.

9. Place a napkin under the patient's chin.

10. Butter the bread and cut up large pieces of meat or vegetables.

    Leave the food and items on the tray in nice order.

11. Place pieces of solid food on the tip of a spoon. Hold the spoon at a right angle.

    Tell and show the patient what kind of food is on the spoon. Test hot foods before feeding them to the patient.

12. Feed the patient in an unhurried manner. Allow the patient to chew the food properly.

13. Offer frequent sips of the fluids provided on the tray. Allow the patient to drink from a straw.

    Do not uncover the hot drink until the patient is ready for it.

14. Encourage the patient to eat and to do as much as possible without help.

    Explain the importance of eating as part of the patient's therapy.

15. Use a napkin or clean face cloth to wipe the mouth as often as needed.

16. Remove the tray as soon as the patient is finished.

17. Record the type and amount of food taken in. If intake and output has been ordered, record the exact amount of fluid the patient drank.

    If the patient could not eat or refused to eat, report this to the charge nurse.

GIVING A TUBE FEEDING

A tube feeding is one given through a nasogastric tube. One end of the tube remains outside the nose and the other rests in the stomach. This is a method to give nourishment when the patient cannot be fed by mouth. The nourishment given through the tube is in the form of a thick liquid. The liquid contains many nutrients and provides a balanced diet for the patient. This liquid provides a richer nourishment than that pro-vided through I.V. fluids. Some conditions permit patients to receive nourishment only through I.V. fluids. However, whenever possible, the richer tube feedings are started. Tube feedings are discontinued when the patient can take food by mouth.

PROCEDURE

1. Assemble equipment:

    Emesis basin
    Bulb syringe
    500 ml graduate measure
    Cotton drawsheet
    Solution bowl with warm water 105°F (40.5°C)
    Tissue wipes
    Feeding as ordered

2. Greet patient and explain procedure.

3. Screen the unit.

4. Place the feeding in a basin of warm water. The feeding should be lukewarm.

5. Place the patient in Fowler's position. Drape the patient's shoulders with a cotton drawsheet.

    If the patient cannot tolerate the position, the dorsal recumbent position may be used.

6. Remove the clamp from the nasogastric tube and attach the syringe to tube.

    The tube is clamped when not in use to prevent air from entering the stomach.

7. Determine that the tube is in the stomach by withdrawing a small amount of the stomach contents with the syringe.

    Check to see that the tube is not in the trachea. Putting fluid into the trachea could block the airway.

8. Remove the bulb from the syringe and put the bulb aside.

9. Pour 30 ml (1 ounce) warm water through the syringe and allow it to run by gravity to flush the tube.

   If water does not run through the tube easily, call the supervising nurse or doctor to check it. Do not exert pressure.

10. Allow prescribed amount of feeding to run in slowly by gravity. The amount usually given is 150 ml (5 ounces). However, the maximum should not exceed 500 ml (16 1/2 ounces) per feeding.

    Rate of flow may be increased by raising the syringe or decreased by lowering it. The flow should be about 20 ml (2/3 ounces) per minute. Keep the syringe filled to prevent air from entering the stomach.

11. Flush tube with 30 ml (1 ounce) of warm water after the feeding but before the syringe has emptied.

    To prevent the introduction of air bubbles.

12. Replace clamp. Secure the tube to patient's clothing or the pillow case.

    When tube is retained for several days, special oral hygiene should be given frequently. The nostrils should be

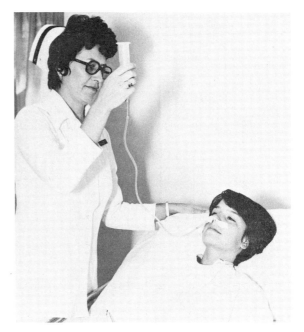

Fig. 73-1 Nourishment should be given in a relaxed, unhurried manner.

lubricated to prevent crusts from forming.

13. Assist the patient back into a comfortable position. Encourage the patient to rest after the feeding.

14. Clean the syringe, wrap it in a clean towel and leave it near the bedside.

15. Record the type and the amount of feeding given on the intake and output sheet. Record this in the patient's chart. Note the time and the patient's reaction to the tube feeding.

VOCABULARY

- Define the following words:

  balanced diet   nourishment

SUGGESTED ACTIVITIES

- Ask another student to role play as a patient. Prepare a food tray with a well balanced diet and practice feeding it to the patient. After the meal, discuss with the student whether the meal was relaxing. Evaluate your technique.

- Obtain permission to visit the diet kitchen in a local hospital. Observe the dietician's staff preparing tube feedings. Inquire as to which nutrients are included in the nourishment solution.

REVIEW

Briefly answer the following questions.

1. What information does the label on a food tray include?

2. Why is the tube feeding placed in a basin of water before being given?

3. What is the usual amount of fluid given in one tube feeding?

4. Why is it necessary to lubricate the nostrils of a patient who has a naso-gastric tube inserted?

5. Give two reasons why the nurse should use an unhurried manner in feeding a patient.

unit 74 care of the aging

OBJECTIVES

After studying this unit, the student will be able to:

- Explain the changes which occur during the process of aging.
- Identify the special nursing care techniques needed for the aged.

Aging is usually a slow, gradual process. The age of sixty-five has been mistakenly accepted as the time for the onset of old age. This may have resulted from the fact that sixty-five is commonly the age for retirement. Each person undergoes the aging process at a different rate. Health as well as personal differences determine whether a patient feels old. The nurse should avoid making assumptions about aged patients. Some patients at eighty are more active and alert than patients who are fifty.

PHYSIOLOGICAL CHANGES IN AGING

Geriatrics is the study and treatment of diseases of aging. The process of aging is accompanied by many physical changes in the body. Bones become brittle and break easily. Injuries also heal more slowly in the aged. The patient's skin becomes thin and dry and is more easily irritated. This skin condition allows bedsores to form if proper care is not given. Deformities are also more likely to occur since muscles become less elastic. The aging process also may suppress the senses. Hearing and vision commonly become less acute.

Poor nutrition and decreased fluid intake often become problems for the aged. Poor nutrition usually results from a patient's loss of appetite. This may be due to a number of causes. If the patient's teeth are loose or missing, chewing food is difficult. Lack of

mouth care also reduces appetite. Patients living at home who do not enjoy cooking or eating alone rarely eat regular meals. Poor nutrition may result from dependence on a few select foods. The patient's poor eating practices often reflect lifetime habits.

Drinking the proper amount of fluids can also be difficult for some patients. Physical changes often depress the sensation of thirst. Thirst normally acts as a guide in maintaining fluid balance. Insufficient fluid intake can lead to constipation and kidney problems.

Nursing Care

The nurse can help reduce the problems caused by physical changes in the aged.

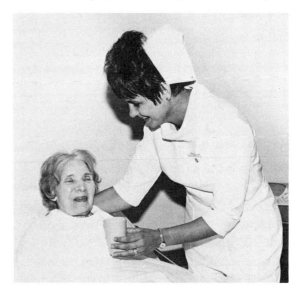

Fig. 74-1 Fluid intake may need to be encouraged.

Frequent change of position and increased activity within the patient's limits are essential. This helps to stimulate circulation, prevent deformity and decubiti, and maintain muscle tone. Massage will benefit circulation. Devices such as the footboard and bed cradle may be helpful in preventing deformities. They keep the weight of bedcovers from falling on the patient's limbs disturbing proper alignment. Skin care is important in preventing decubiti. If a break in the skin occurs, it must be reported immediately. Care must be taken to prevent sores and infections. Keeping the patient's skin clean and applying lotions to keep it soft helps to keep it healthy.

PSYCHOLOGICAL CHANGES IN AGING

The process of aging does not change the needs people develop throughout life. The aged, like the young, need security, love, recognition and a sense of purpose. Many problems of aging disrupt the fulfillment of these needs. Physical changes often cause psychological changes. Illness and physical disorders may require patients to depend on others for their care. Many people resent the need to ask for help with bathing, feeding and toileting. Those who require this care permanently may need to leave their homes. This can isolate the patient from people who provide needed love and security. The change also separates the patient from familiar surroundings.

Nursing Care

The nurse must show concern for the patient's emotional problems as well as the physical problems. The patient is often helped by knowing the nurse cares. Physical problems can sometimes be reduced through services provided by other health team members. A physical therapist or dietician, for example, can work with the nurse to improve the con-

dition of some patients. The nurse should also provide the patient with a chance to attend religious services. Counseling from a minister, priest or rabbi may also provide great comfort for the patient.

Planning activities that interest the patient is needed in the hospital or the nursing home. Allowing patients to eat together often improves the appetite. It also makes mealtime more pleasant. Group activities, hobbies, reading or watching television all can provide enjoyment. Social involvement usually improves the patient's attitude. Emotional health helps the patient cope with physical problems.

MENTAL CONFUSION

Confused behavior in the aged is often due to a physical disorder. Confusion may be temporary and involve only forgetfulness. However, a confused patient also may be unable to speak or reason clearly.

Physical changes in the arteries may block circulation to the brain. This leads to permanent damage in the brain. Confusion may also occur with *senile brain atrophy*. In this condition some of the nerve cells die. Usually these conditions worsen gradually. Another type of confusion may result from a mental breakdown. This occurs because the patient is unable to cope with a specific stress. Loss of loved ones, loss of self-image or various other factors can create stress in the aged.

Nursing Care

The nurse can usually help comfort the confused patient, no matter what the cause. Some patients respond well to *orientation therapy*. This is a method used to stimulate the senses. It also involves reminding the patient of the date and the time repeatedly. This technique, also called reality orientation, helps the patient communicate with others.

The nurse can help the confused patient by speaking in a direct manner. Being consistent and keeping routines helps reduce the stress of change.

VOCABULARY

- Define the following words:

    brittle   reality orientation   retirement
    emotional   recognition   senile brain atrophy
    geriatrics

SUGGESTED ACTIVITIES

- Mr. J. has recently been admitted to the hospital for diagnosis. Many tests have been planned in order to make the diagnosis. Mr. J. shows signs of being depressed. He comments that all of his friends have died in recent years and that no one at home understands him. Prepare a care plan for him during his stay in the hospital which will lessen his depression.

- Study and discuss the uses of reality orientation.

REVIEW

Select the *best* answer.

1. The aging process progresses

    a. after the age of sixty-five
    b. after retirement
    c. at a different rate for each person
    d. when a patient enters a nursing home

2. The term which describes the study and treatment for diseases of aging is

    a. geriatrics   c. senility
    b. pediatrics   d. confusion

3. Loss of appetite usually results from

    a. poor condition of the teeth   c. lack of enjoyment in eating
    b. poor mouth care   d. all of the above

4. Increasing the activity level of an aged patient helps

    a. prevent senile brain atrophy
    b. reduce the need for security
    c. prevent decubiti and maintain muscle tone
    d. prevent physiological changes in aging

5. The nurse can help the patient preserve emotional health by

    a. sending patients home from the hospital early
    b. planning activities that interest the patient
    c. serving meals in the hall instead of the room
    d. comparing personal problems with those of the patient

unit 75 care of the dying patient

OBJECTIVES

After studying this unit, the student will be able to:

- Describe ways to assist a patient when death is imminent.

- List the items often used by the priest to perform the sacrament of the sick.

Nurses have a unique role in helping a patient who is close to death. A major part of this care is helping the family through that time of crisis. A nurse who has dealt with the patient or the family earlier can be of great comfort. People differ widely in their ability to cope with feelings about death. Therefore, the nurse cannot assume how the patient or the family will feel. The nurse should be aware of both the patient's physical and spiritual needs. Patients close to death are placed on a critically ill list. In some states, the law requires that the hospital notify the family and a member of the clergy.

Many patients seek spiritual help during the last critical period of life. The nurse should inform the patient that religious counselors and clergy are available. Visits of this kind can provide great comfort to the patient and family. Even though death may have been expected, the final hours bring a special crisis point.

The nurse should be aware of the specific faith professed by the dying patient. Certain religious faiths dictate rituals which must be followed just prior to death or soon after. Members of the Jewish or Protestant faith may need no special practice performed before death. However, the nurse may be asked to read a spiritual passage or share a prayer with the patient. The patient may require only that the nurse stay near and be a caring listener. The nurse does not always have the same beliefs as the patient but she should nevertheless show respect and concern.

Roman Catholics believe in receiving the sacrament of the sick before death. The sacrament of the sick can provide strength and comfort to the sick or dying patient. The patient may wish to have a confession heard by a priest at this time. The family may be present at the sacrament of the sick except for the time the confession is heard by the priest.

If a Roman Catholic has reached the critical stage without having received the sacrament of the sick, a priest should be called. The nurse should be sure the priest has the items needed to perform the sacrament. Some health facilities have sets of these items available for use. Also, the priest may bring many of the items with him. The nurse should check the policy of the health facility to determine which items are needed. The following articles should be placed on a small clean table just before the priest is expected.

Crucifix

Container with cotton balls

Clean folded towel

Two candle holders and two wax candles candles which have been blessed

Matches

Other items which may be needed but are usually brought by the priest are:

Sprinkler bottle of holy water

Small amount of salt in a container in which the tip of the thumb can be inserted.

Oils

Communion bread

The nurse will quietly withdraw from the bedside when the priest, minister, or rabbi arrives. The curtains may be drawn slightly for added privacy until the departure of the clergyman. Remember to chart the visit. Meeting spiritual needs — as well as physical and psychological needs — is part of nursing care.

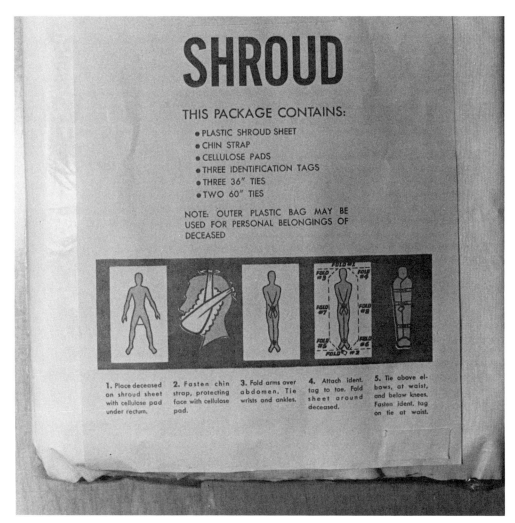

Fig. 75-1 The shroud package label instructs the nurse how to prepare the body after death.

VOCABULARY

- Define the following words:

clergy	crucifix	Roman Catholic
confession	Jewish	sacrament
counselor	Protestant	spiritual
crisis	ritual	

SUGGESTED ACTIVITY

- Investigate and report to the class on the various religious practices that a nurse may need to know in professional practice.

REVIEW

Select the *best* answer.

1. Receiving the sacrament of the sick is practiced by
   - a. Protestants
   - b. Roman Catholics
   - c. Mennonites
   - d. Jews

2. The nurse can sometimes help the patient cope with impending death by
   - a. reading a spiritual passage
   - b. sharing a prayer with the patient
   - c. being an attentive listener
   - d. all of the above

3. To gather items for the priest in performing the sacrament of the sick, the nurse should first
   - a. check the policy of the health facility
   - b. ask the patient what items are needed
   - c. ask the family to leave the patient's room
   - d. ask a Roman Catholic nurse to get the items

4. An important part of assisting the dying patient is
   - a. reading long bible passages aloud
   - b. isolating the dying patient from the family
   - c. helping the patient's family
   - d. telling the patient about your own beliefs

5. The nurse should not impose personal beliefs on the patient or family because
   - a. people differ widely in the way they view death
   - b. people without religious faith usually do not want comforting
   - c. patients who have had long illnesses do not feel the crisis
   - d. the nurse should avoid showing concern for the patient

SELF-EVALUATION XII

A. Select the *best* answer.

1. An advantage of the Stryker frame is that

    a. no lifting is required to place the patient on the bedpan
    b. the patient can feed himself in the prone position
    c. the patient can be turned and transported easily
    d. all of the above

2. Before turning a patient in a Stryker frame, the patient should

    a. have a complete bed bath
    b. sign a consent slip
    c. be given an explanation of how it works
    d. be weighed

3. The special bed which can be used to support the patient in a weight bearing position is the

    a. Circle® bed   c. traction apparatus
    b. Stryker frame   d. all of the above

4. A patient in a stupor may react to unpleasant stimuli by

    a. retracting   c. making a groaning sound
    b. grimacing   d. all of the above

5. Incontinence means

    a. genitourinary tract infection
    b. painful sensation with urination
    c. loss of control over elimination of urine or feces
    d. excretion of body wastes

6. Special care used to prevent decubiti includes

    a. keeping the patient on bedrest as long as possible
    b. turning the patient in bed frequently
    c. moistening folds in the skin
    d. all of the above

7. The indwelling catheter is ordered

    a. whenever intake and output is recorded
    b. whenever fluid intake is increased
    c. to keep an incontinent patient clean and dry
    d. to relieve constipation

8. When feeding a patient, the spoon is held

   a. straight
   b. at a right angle
   c. pointing upward
   d. in the left hand

9. Nasogastric tube feedings are used to

   a. irrigate the stomach
   b. provide nourishment when a patient cannot take food orally
   c. aid the patient in breathing
   d. administer I.V. fluids

10. Careless handling when suctioning a patient with a tracheostomy may

    a. cause trauma to the tissue
    b. increase secretions
    c. raise the possibility of infection
    d. all of the above

11. Poor nutrition in the aged may result from

    a. a poor appetite
    b. old age syndrome
    c. overactivity
    d. not taking vitamin supplements

12. Care of the unconscious patient includes

    a. carefully observing and recording the patient's condition
    b. turning the patient frequently
    c. providing good skin care
    d. all of the above

13. The nurse can determine if a nasogastric tube is in the stomach by

    a. blowing on the opposite end of the tube
    b. forcing 100 ml (3 ounces) of water into the tube
    c. leaving the tube unclamped to observe drainage
    d. withdrawing some of the gastric contents

14. Confused behavior in the aged may be due to a disorder which is

    a. physiological
    b. temporary
    c. permanent
    d. all of the above

15. Incontinence can be caused by

    a. unconsciousness
    b. decubiti
    c. poor skin care
    d. regular emptying of the bladder

B. Match the term in column II with the description in column I.

Column I

_____ 1. surgical opening made into the trachea
_____ 2. provides nourishment for patients who cannot eat by mouth
_____ 3. part of the tracheostomy tube removed only by a doctor
_____ 4. equipment which supports and rotates the body
_____ 5. study of diseases of aging
_____ 6. an unconscious state
_____ 7. to inhale material into the trachea
_____ 8. medications which help regulate the bowel
_____ 9. religious act performed for the dying patient
_____ 10. reminding the patient of the date and the time repeatedly

Column II

a. tracheostomy
b. tilt table
c. sacrament of the sick
d. orientation therapy
e. cathartics
f. outer cannula
g. inner cannula
h. aspirate
i. inhalation therapist
j. esophageal speech
k. coma
l. tube feeding
m. geriatrics
n. senile brain atrophy

APPENDIX: Learning Medical Terms

OBJECTIVES

After studying this unit, the student will be able to:

- Define roots, prefixes and suffixes commonly used in medical terms.

- Give the meaning of abbreviations commonly used in giving health care.

Learning medical terminology at times seems to be a difficult task. However, if the student studies a few words at a time, the process becomes easier. Medical terms can also be broken down in order to speed learning. To do this, it is necessary to master a few prefixes, suffixes and roots. A *prefix* is the term given to letters or syllables united with the beginning of a word. A *suffix* refers to letters or syllables united with the end of a word. A *root* is the main part of the word to which the prefix or suffix is added.

Common prefixes, suffixes, roots and abbreviations will become a part of the student's working vocabulary. For example, the prefix *hydro* refers to water and the word *therapy* means treatment. Thus, *hydrotherapy* means treatment with water. The suffix *itis* means inflammation of. Therefore, when the term *tonsilitis* is used, it means inflammation of the tonsils. The root *nephro* refers to the kidneys. The word *nephritis* means inflammation of the kidneys.

PREFIXES

(United with the beginning of a word)

a–, an–	without or decreased	ecto–	outside
ab–	away from	en–	in, into
adeno–	gland, glandular	endo–	inside
ante–	before	epi–	upon
auto–	self	ex–, exo–	out, away from
bi–, bis–	twice, double	glyco–	sugar
bili–	bile	gynec–	woman
centi–	hundred, hundredth	hecto–	one hundred
contra–	against	hem–, hemo–	blood
cysto–, cyst–	like a bag or bladder	hepato–	liver
de–	from	homo–	same, similar
demi–	half	hydro–	water
dis–	not, apart, absence of	hyper–	above, high
		hypo–	below, under
dorso–	back, to the back	inter–	between
dys–	bad, difficult	intra–	within

iso–	equal	pluri–	more, several
leuco–, leuko–	white	post–	after
mal–	poor, bad	pre–	before
macro–	large	proto–	first
micro–	small	pseudo–	false
mono–	one, single	pyo–	related to pus
multi–	many	retro–	backward
neo–	new	semi–	half
neur–, neuro–	nerve	sub–	under
non–	not	super–, supra–	above
ob–	against	syn–	with, together
ortho–	straight, correction	thermo–	heat
pan–	entire	trans–	across
para–	beside, accessory to	tri–	three
patho–	disease	ventro–	to the front, abdomen
peri–	around		

SUFFIXES
(United with the ending of a word)

–algia	pain	–osis	disease, condition
–cele	swelling, tumor	–ous	full of
–cide	causing death	–oxy	sharp, acid
–cyst	bladder, bag	–pathy	suffering, abnormal feeling
–cyte	cell		
–ectomy	surgical removal	–penia	lack
–emia	blood	–phobia	fear
–gen, –genesis	production	–plastic	molded
–gram	tracing, record	–plegia	stroke
–graph	writing, recording	–ptosis	falling
–itis	inflammation	–rhage, –ragia	excessive flow
–ize	to treat with	–rhapy	suturing
–lysis	setting free disintegration	–rhea	discharge
		–stomy	to furnish with an opening
–meter	measure		
–ode, –oid	resembling resemblance to	–trophic	relating to nourishment
–ology	study of	–tropic	turning
–oma	tumor	–uria	relating to urine

ROOTS
(Form the base of a word)

Root	Pertains to	Root	Pertains to
adeno	glands	cardio	heart
arthro	joints	dermato	skin

Root	Pertains to	Root	Pertains to
gastro	stomach	osteo	bone or bones
meno	menstruation	phlebo	vein or veins
myo	muscle or muscles	psyche	mind
nephro	kidney or kidneys	thoraco	chest
neuro	nerve or nerves		

ABBREVIATIONS

Abbreviation	Meaning	Abbreviation	Meaning
a.c.	before meals	o.m.	every morning
ad lib.	as much as desired	o.n.	every night
aq.	water	oz.	ounce
aq. dest.	distilled water	p.c.	after meals
b.i.d.	twice a day	p.r.n.	when necessary
B.P.	blood pressure	q.d.	every day
°C.	Celsius	q.h.	every hour
c	with	q.i.d.	four times a day
Cal.	calorie (standard)	q.s.	sufficient quantity
cm³	cubic centimeter	s	without
et	and	sig.	give with following
F.	Fahrenheit		directions
gm	gram	s.o.s.	if necessary
gr.	grain	ss	one half
Gtt., gtt.	a drop, drops	stat.	immediately
h	hour	t.i.d.	three times a day
h.s.	at bedtime	T.P.R.	temperature, pulse,
I.V.	intravenously		respiration
o.d.	daily	tsp.	teaspoon
o.l.	every hour	WBC	white blood cell count

OPTIONAL REVIEW

A. Make a list of five medical terms using a prefix or suffix in each term. Underline the prefix or suffix. Then, using a medical dictionary, give the meaning of the term.

Example: Claustro<u>phobia</u> – fear of being enclosed

B. Match the term in Column I with the definition in Column II. Look for the prefix or suffix to help clarify the meaning of the term.

Column I	Column II
_____ 1. neuralgia	a. surgical removal of appendix
_____ 2. hypertension	b. inflammation of a joint
_____ 3. pyuria	c. excessive bleeding
_____ 4. hemorrhage	d. treatment using water
_____ 5. arthritis	e. form of mental illness
_____ 6. hydrotherapy	f. pus in the urine
_____ 7. appendectomy	g. pain in a nerve
_____ 8. phlebitis	h. high blood pressure
_____ 9. paraplegia	i. inflammation of the bladder
_____ 10. psychosis	j. false labor
	k. paralysis of the legs
	l. inflamed vein

C. Draw a slash through the following terms to separate the root from the prefix or suffix. Give the meaning of each word using a medical dictionary.

Example: Meno/pause — period marking the end of menstrual activity

1. Bilious

2. Colostomy

3. Dystrophy

4. Hyperglycemia

5. Hypodermic

6. Leukocyte

7. Myoma

8. Gynecology

9. Septicemia

10. Atrophic

ACKNOWLEDGMENTS

The author would like to thank the following for their services and cooperation.

Mrs. Carol A. Seeley, RN, BA, Director of Nurses, Silver Haven Nursing Home, Schenectady, New York, for use of their facilities

B. Blair Brooks for some of the photographs

Justine Hodges, Katherine Owen, Erwin G. Simmons and Esther G. Skelley for their assistance in the preparation of the original text.

Each person who consented to be a subject in the photographs

Rockingham Community College, Wentworth, N.C. for permission to use the photograph on the title page

The author also wishes to thank the following companies for the illustrations.

American Hospital Supply, figures 32-4, 55-1, 70-3

Baxter Laboratories Inc., figure 29-2

Burron Medical Products, figure 11-1

Dison, Norma G. *An Atlas of Nursing Techniques.* ed. 2, C.V. Mosby Co., figure 30-1

Eli Lilly and Co., figure 25-2

Gomco Surgical Manufacturing Co., figure 57-1

Gormann-Rupp Industries, figure 50-1

Hollister, Inc., figure 65-1

IVAC Corp., figure 13-1

Kendall, Hospital Products Division, figure 18-1

Linde Division, Union Carbide Corp., figure 58-3

Metropolitan Life Insurance Co., figure 23-1

Mueller, V., figure 69-1

Stryker Corp., figures 9-2, 70-1

Contributions by Delmar Staff

Sponsoring Editor — Angela R. Emmi

Source Editor — Anne Greatbatch

INDEX

9/88(7C1966I)